Natural Beauty Basics

Natural Beauty Basics

CREATE YOUR OWN COSMETICS AND BODY CARE PRODUCTS

Dorie Byers, R.N.

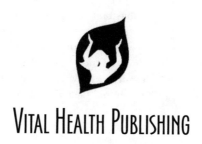

VITAL HEALTH PUBLISHING

Natural Beauty Basics:
Make Your Own Cosmetics and Body Care Products
Dorie Byers, R.N.

Second edition copyright ©2001 Dorie Byers
Second Printing, 2005
All rights reserved.
Originally published as *Natural Body Basics: Making Your Own Cosmetics,*
1996, Gooseberry Hill Publications.

Printed in the United States of America by Versa Press, Inc.,
East Peoria, IL.

Text Design by Studio 2D, Champaign, IL.
Cover Design by On The Dot Designs, Austin, TX.
Illustrations by Susan Cavaciuti.

Vital Health Publishing
34 Mill Plain Road
Danbury, CT 06811
www.vitalhealthbooks.com

ISBN: 1-890612-19-7

DISCLAIMER
The author and publisher have made every effort to ensure the accuracy and completeness of information in this book. We assume no responsibility for errors, inaccuracies, omissions, or any inconsistency herein.

The safe and proper use of all ingredients and any of the recipes in this book is the sole responsibility of the person(s) using them. The author and publisher are not responsible for any misuse or carelessness by the user. Likewise, the author and publisher are not responsible for any allergic reactions. None of the advice in this book should be mistaken for medical advice. Any concerns about any condition the user may have should be addressed by a professional medical practitioner.

§

Thanks to my husband Rick and son Jason for their help, love, and support. This work wouldn't have been possible if it weren't for you both. Special thanks to Jim for the encouragement. And thanks to Sway, my best tester and critic. I hope you all enjoy my effort. Love to you all.

Contents

Preface

Taking care of yourself means making *healthy* choices. A dizzying number of ads tells us on a daily basis that we cannot have a pleasing and healthy appearance without buying and using numerous commercial products. The fact is that we can attain a healthy appearance without the purchase of these products and be more in control over our well-being besides.

Making body care products out of natural ingredients provides us with an alternative to commercial preparations. A *glowing appearance* can still be the end result when using products with recognizable ingredients.

When the cost of making your own body care products is calculated, significant monetary savings should be noticed as well. Add up the cost of your ingredients and figure out the amount of product you can make. Make a comparison of the cost of an equal quantity of commercial products that are advertised to achieve a similar result on your body. It is my opinion that you will be quite pleased with the savings that you will realize by making your own body care products.

When making recipes for natural cosmetics found in a variety of books and magazine articles, I have generally been disappointed by the finished product. My reaction to these disappointments has been to experiment with combining various ingredients on my own. After doing some personal research and trying different combinations of ingredients, I have come up with many recipes containing natural ingredients that you can make with a little effort. All the information you need is contained in this book.

It is well documented and important to remember that many people suffer from allergic and/or sensitivity reactions to chemical additives in commercial cosmetics. Two examples are synthetic fragrances and parabens. Synthetic fragrances can cause headaches, dizziness, rash, and/or skin irritations in susceptible individuals. Parabens (methyl, propyl, butyl, and ethyl) are used to inhibit microbial growth to extend the shelf life of products, and can cause skin rashes. Replacing these and any other synthetic ingredients for natural ingredients to achieve the results that you want can be helpful in cases where allergies and sensitivities are an issue. The "Guide to Ingredients" section and the recipes throughout this book can give you a multitude of alternatives to commercial products that you are unable to use.

Enjoy exploring this natural, healing knowledge. Here's to your well-being!

&Introduction

There are many body care products available commercially but when you go to the store to make your choices, it turns into a real challenge. Reading the labels adds to the puzzle. It seems that we need a college degree in chemistry just to understand the ingredients. We don't actually know what we are putting on our skin and hair and absorbing into our bodies.

Did you ever price cosmetics in a department store? In general, the prices of these commercial products really amaze me. A small tube of high quality hand cream can cost from $3 to $12 – even at a drug or discount store! Specialized products for the hair and body can cost more than that. If products are purchased at a cosmetics counter in a major department store the price will likely be much higher. Read the label on any product that you are thinking of purchasing. The ingredients listed first on any label signify that they comprise the greatest percentage of the total composition of the product. Commonly you will find that the first ingredients listed on body care products are water, mineral oil, alcohol, or witch hazel. None of these ingredients by themselves are expensive. Also, some of these ingredients are not necessarily helpful in certain situations. Alcohol and witch hazel can be too drying for some skin types, while mineral oil has large molecules and can clog the skin's pores. None of these ingredients alone are expensive, but when the manufacturer figures in the cost of packaging, advertising, other additives, and their overhead, the price increases significantly.

Now go to a natural foods store and read the labels on body care products. The ingredients listed on the labels are more understandable in most cases, but the price remains high. A jar of herbal deodorant cream is $14.95! A tube of face mask costs $11, and the ingredients are clay and an herbal infusion. For the price of the tube of face mask, a container of clay and a package of dried herbs could be purchased to make face masks enough to easily last six months, and still have money left over. If the herb I chose to use for the infusion was one that grows in my garden, then the total price would decrease even more.

Making your own natural cosmetics is not only economical, but can be beneficial to your skin. The best part about making your own cosmetics is that, with a bit of research and using ingredients available, you can custom-make your products to suit your own skin's needs. You can substitute one natural ingredient for another to meet your individual requirements and preferences. The results can be as satisfactory as those achieved from commercial products. There are no artificial ingredients, so the mystery of what is being put on your skin and absorbed into your body is absent.

It can be a very satisfying activity to make your own body care products. Most recipes are as simple a making cookies from scratch. I feel a sense of contentment when seeing little jars and pots of creams and powders that I make sitting on the bathroom shelf. It makes me feel good to have control over another step toward a healthier life. I know exactly what is in each container, that the products are freshly made, and what it cost to make each one. I also know what it doesn't have—chemicals with unpronounceable names and a high price tag. When allergies and sensitivities to chemical additives are a problem, the recipes in this book provide a healthy alternative. Those who still want to use cosmetics can make their own products with satisfying results and no risk of contact with ingredients that cause negative reactions to them.

Homemade body care products provide a humane alternative to commercial ones, alleviating the concerns of vegetarians and animal lovers among my readers. None of the ingredients contain animal by-products, nor have any of the recipes been tested on animals.

Making your own cosmetics is versatile. Products can be individualized for yourself, your family, and friends regardless of gender or age. Custom made gift giving is easy if you know the skin type of any given individual. If you don't have that information, make a general skin care product such as body oil, powder, or soap. It will be a welcome gift that will be used with pleasure.

It is fun experimenting with all of the ingredients available to you. Be creative and use the different sections of this book as your reference guides to make a recipe of your very own.

Equipment

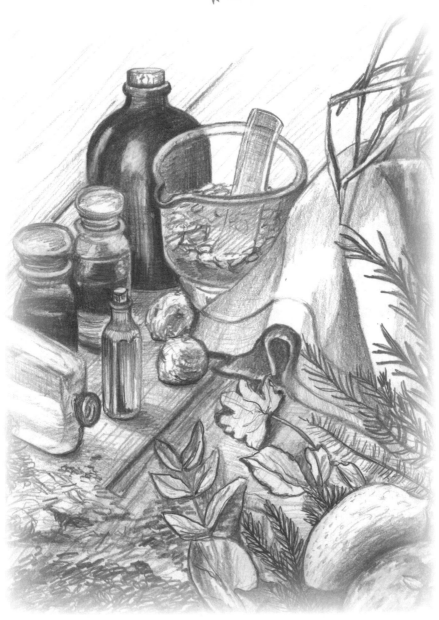

$\mathcal{S}$earch through your kitchen cabinets and drawers for the supplies required to make the recipes in this book. Here are the basics.

ESSENTIALS

Clean needle

A common sewing needle cleaned with soap and water and then dried may be used to obtain the contents of gelcaps containing Vitamin E or evening primrose oil.

Double boiler

Choose an enamelware or stainless steel one. If you don't have a double boiler, try the following arrangement, which works well for me. Place a heat proof glass bowl or measuring cup in a saucepan with two to three inches of boiling water in it, then mix and prepare your recipe as recommended in the glass container.

Eyedroppers

Glass eyedroppers are preferable and should be available to use with essential oils if the essential oil bottles don't have a built-in dropper. Keep several on hand, so that you will have one eye dropper for each essential oil bottle used when making a recipe. Wash and dry eye droppers thoroughly before using in another essential oil bottle to prevent the accidental mixing of the essential oils, keeping each individual essential oil pure.

Note: in the "old days" the bulbs of eye droppers were made of natural rubber, but now they are made from synthetic substances that can leach potentially toxic materials into any liquids put into contact with them. Do not overfill eyedroppers so that the liquids come into contact with the bulb, and do not leave eyedroppers in the bottles where the cosmetic ingredients are stored to avoid contact with any of these materials.

Flour sifter

Food processor, blender, or electric coffee grinder

Any of these will work fine to grind seeds, grains, nuts, and dried plant material into very small powder-like particles.

Funnel, small to medium sized

Glass jars and bottles

If you have them available, brown or amber glass is best to help keep products from deteriorating due to exposure to light. Recycle extract bottles, baby food jars, and large mouth jars of all kinds. Plastic containers are adequate, but will soak up the odor of anything that is placed in them, and it is impossible to eliminate those odors. Also the extracts or preparations themselves will absorb small amounts of the plastic container gradually over time.

I suggest asking friends to save glass containers for you. I have frequently recruited the mothers of infants to save baby food jars for me. Before using, make sure that any recycled containers are thoroughly washed and dried. (To obtain new containers, see the Resources section in the back of this book.)

Photographic or illustrated herb identification book

Your resource must have detailed plant descriptions and pictures to make positive identification possible. My favorite is *Rodale's Illustrated Encyclopedia of Herbs* published by Rodale Press. (See the Bibliography in the back of this book for further information.) You can also browse in a book store for a resource that suits your needs, or ask someone who is well-versed in herbs for a recommendation.

Well-written reference book for essential oils and aromatherapy

For more detailed information on the use of essential oils and the art of aromatherapy, obtain a book that is solely based on the subject. There are many available, but my current favorite is *Aromatherapy: A Lifetime Guide to Healing with Essential Oils* by Valerie Gennari Cooksley. (See the

Bibliography in the back of this book for further information.) You can also seek the advice of a trained aromatherapist for suggestions.

Grater

Get an old grater you've picked up at a garage sale or one that you no longer use for food preparation. Some ingredients that require grating, like beeswax, are nearly impossible to remove from a grater.

Heat proof glass measuring cups

For most recipes, a one cup measure will be adequate.

Hot pads or oven mitts

These are essential to protect you from burns when handling hot containers and ingredients.

Mortar and pestle

This equipment can be used to grind or crush herbs or seeds into smaller sizes. If you don't own a mortar and pestle, you can always place whatever it is that you want to crush on a cutting board, cover it with plastic wrap, and hit it several times with a rolling pin. (This also helps to release any negative feelings that might be bothering you!)

Paper coffee filters

One of these is placed in a strainer or sieve to prevent any small particles from passing into the finished product. Use the brown unbleached filters if possible.

Reusable muslin tea bags

These small bags with a drawstring are ideal to hold herbs for bath bag mixtures or herbal infusions. If you can't find them or don't want to purchase any, a clean sock that no longer has a mate can be pressed into service. Either of these can be easily washed and dried to be used over and over again.

Saucepan, stainless steel or enamelware

A small or medium sized saucepan is all that you should need. Depending on the ingredients used, cookware made from materials other than stainless steel or enamelware has the ability to leach elements into some mixtures, changing the composition of the finished product.

Soap molds

Certain soap recipes use molds to form the finished product into desired shapes. These can be purchased from soap-making supply companies. Small dishes or other containers commonly found in the kitchen can be used as soap molds. Any container to be used as a soap mold must have the tops wider than the bottoms, otherwise the finished product is impossible to remove. Plastic containers can retain the fragrance of essential oils which is almost impossible to remove, so keep this in mind before using any of your kitchen containers as soap molds. Clean 8-ounce yogurt cups can be used as disposable soap molds. Cut the sides of the cups down until the cup is 1-2 inches deep before using. (For companies that sell soap molds, see the Resources section in the back of this book.)

Spatula

There are new heat-resistant ones make of silicone that I like to use instead of rubber or plastic ones. If you don't have the heat-resistant silicone ones, then keep the exposure of extremely hot substances to a minimum with the rubber or plastic spatulas.

Standard measuring cups and spoons

Keep a variety of sizes on hand.

Strainer or sieve, small

Wire whisk

A smaller sized one works best, but a large one will do if that is what you have available.

Guide to Ingredients

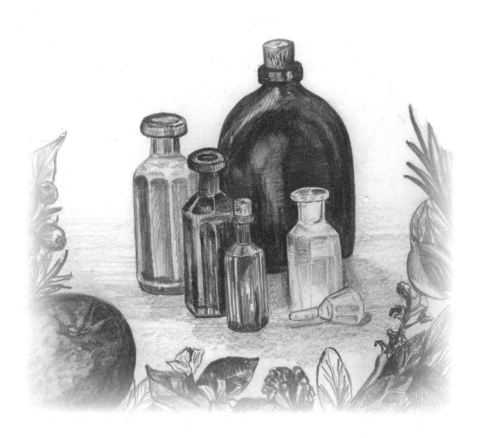

This guide contains information about individual ingredients. It may also be used as a reference when customizing recipes to meet your specific body care needs.

SPECIAL INFORMATION
CONCERNING INGREDIENTS

❦ *Read all labels before making a purchase to be sure that you are buying the correct item(s).*

❦ *Buy organic ingredients, if available, to avoid unnecessary contact with pesticides or herbicides which are not eliminated during processing.*

❦ *Look for cold-pressed or low heat processed oils that contain no preservatives and are not extracted with solvents.*

❦ *Store ingredients containing oils in the refrigerator to prolong shelf life. Nuts and seeds contain oil as a natural part of their makeup and should be refrigerated or frozen as well.*

Almond – A nut used, finely ground, as an ingredient for facial scrubs.

Aloe Vera Gel – A clear gel obtained from the inside of the leaves of the *Aloe vera* plant. Used in hair care and skin care, the gel has healing and emollient properties. Look for the least processed gel available. Avoid buying gel that has artificial coloring added.

Apricot Kernel Oil – A clear golden-colored oil that has a light feel and is useful to soften all skin types. It may be used full strength on the skin.

Arrowroot Powder – A fine white powder obtained from the root of the plant *Maranta arundincea*. It is used as an ingredient in body powders.

Avocado Oil – A very rich green-gold oil derived from the large seeds of the avocado fruit. This oil absorbs readily into the skin, and is good for all skin types. It is especially effective when used on dry, aged, and/or undernourished skin. It may be used full strength.

Baking Soda – A powdery white substance with deodorizing properties that is used as an addition to body powders.

Beeswax – Naturally golden colored and honey scented solid wax made by bees, it is used as an emulsifier in preparations. It forms a natural protective barrier on the skin, helping to keep moisture from escaping and preventing irritating substances from making contact with the skin. To use, grate and measure according to the recipe directions. Some companies sell beeswax in "pearl" form that is easier to measure and eliminates the step of grating. White beeswax is available, but it has been bleached to achieve its color.

Bentonite – A white-to-gray colored clay that is derived from volcanic ash. Highly absorbent, it is used in face masks and body powders.

Borax – A naturally occurring mineral used as an emulsifier and water softener.

Brewer's Yeast – A byproduct of fermented barley used in beer production. It contains B vitamins and has a very soothing effect on the skin. It is used as an ingredient in face masks.

Castile Soap – A simple soap that contains a vegetable oil as an ingredient. It has a soft foamy lather. Castile soap is available in bar or liquid form.

Castor Oil – A heavy clear oil that is softening to the skin and is rarely linked with allergic reactions. The oil is derived from the beans of *Ricinus communis*. It helps to seal in skin moisture, making it especially beneficial as an ingredient in diaper creams.

Cellulose Chips – Small pieces of plant derived material that will absorb essential oils and 'fix' them for potpourri or sleep pillows. Cellulose chips are usually made of ground corncobs and can be found in pet supply stores sold as bedding.

Cocoa Butter – A creamy white solid wax derived from cacao beans, it is used on the skin to soften and lubricate. Cocoa butter has a pleasant faint chocolate scent. It should be used with caution by people prone to skin allergies.

Coconut Oil – A fine moisturizer derived from fresh coconuts, it is a solid to semi-solid white substance when in a container that liquefies on contact with the warmth of the skin.

Cornmeal – Ground corn used in facial scrubs and soaps.

D-panthenol – This is a naturally occurring form of the B Vitamin pantothenic acid. It is used in shampoo to help the hair feel thicker. There is some evidence that hair absorbs d-panthenol, which gives support from within the hair shaft, making it stronger.

Distilled Water – Water treated by a distillation process, making it free from minerals, chemical impurities, and other substances.

Dried Milk Powder – Milk with the water removed used in baths to soften the skin.

Essential Oils – Highly concentrated essences of herbs added in very small amounts to body care products for aesthetic and/or therapeutic purposes.

Evening Primrose Oil – An oil from the seeds of *Oenothera biennis* that is used as an addition to skin care products. It helps to moisturize dry skin and can be helpful for aging and troubled skin conditions. It is most widely available in gelcaps which can be punctured with a clean needle and the gelcap squeezed to release the oil. Evening primrose oil can also be found in a liquid form that can be measured and used as directed.

Flax Seeds – Seeds from the plant *Linum usitatissimum* that form a gel when soaked in fluid. This gel is softening and moisturizing to the skin, and can be used in face masks.

Fuller's Earth – A naturally occurring clay used in cosmetics and body powders. It absorbs moisture and oil.

Grapefruit Seed Extract – An extract of grapefruit seeds with a glycerine base, its antioxidant properties help prevent cell damage from exposure to free radicals. The extract also has antibacterial properties. It is used as a preservative in body care products, and as an additive in deodorants. Do not use undiluted—it is highly irritating when used full strength.

Grape Seed Oil – A light-textured oil extracted from grape seeds. It absorbs very quickly into the skin, and can be used for any skin type.

Green Clay – Found in the south of France, this clay is pure, mineral-rich, and highly absorbent. It is used in face masks and body powders.

Herbs – Any plant and its part or parts that has a useful purpose to humans, including therapeutic purposes. Depending on the plant, parts used can include flowers, leaves, bark, roots, or seeds.

Honey – A sweet product made by bees used as a skin moisturizer. It can be soothing and healing when applied to troubled skin.

Jasmine Floral Wax – A pliable plant wax that comes from the flowers of *Jasminum grandiflorum*. It is a byproduct from the production of jasmine essential oil. Extremely fragrant, it can be an aromatic moisturizing addition to skin care products.

Jojoba Oil – A naturally occurring liquid wax from the desert plant *Simmondsia chinensis*, it is protective to the skin and helps hair to hold moisture. It can be used as a natural alternative to petroleum jelly. Jojoba oil has an indefinite shelf life. It can be used for all skin types.

Kaolin – Also known as white clay, kaolin is used in face masks and body powders. It absorbs oils and moisture. Its mildly abrasive action can be used in tooth cleaning preparations.

Lanolin – A natural wax that comes from sheep's wool. It is a heavy, thick substance used to protect the skin. It is not recommended for use on oily or very sensitive skin.

Lemon – The sunny yellow fruit whose juice is useful when added to skin or hair products for its antioxidant and astringent properties. It can help to lighten skin and hair and to soften skin, and is deodorizing and cleansing.

Liquid Lecithin – Usually derived from soybeans, lecithin is a natural substance containing Vitamin E, phospholipids, and minerals. It is used as an emulsifier to blend oil-based substances with water-based substances. It is also moisturizing.

Liquid Soap – Any soap product available in liquid form. Read the labels to check for ingredients that are desirable to you. I exclusively use liquid Castile soap that is unscented. Regardless of the type of liquid soap that you buy, always get the unscented brand so that you can add essential oils if you so desire.

Oatmeal – The oat grain rolled flat, used in masks and for bathing. It is an emollient and soothing to the skin.

Olive Oil – A heavy green-gold oil pressed from olives, the fruits of *Olea europaea*. It has a distinctive odor. Olive oil may be used full strength on any skin type, and is very soothing and softening. Buy "extra virgin" olive oil for the highest concentration of vitamins and minerals.

Pure Grain Alcohol – 95% pure alcohol found in liquor stores in some states labeled as "Everclear®". It is used to disperse essential oils and to extract herbal properties from plant parts. Substitute good quality vodka if this substance is not available in your state.

Pure Soap – Soap made without any extra additives as ingredients. Ivory® Soap is an example of pure soap.

Rebatchable Soap Curls – Soap with no other ingredients added other than vegetable oils. It is already shaved or grated and can have any additional ingredients added to it that you desire. The finished product can be shaped into bars or other forms with a few simple steps.

Rosehip Seed Oil – This oil is from the seeds of the rosehips that form after roses (*Rosa* spp.) bloom. Its high Vitamin C and fatty acid content makes it rejuvenating, softening, and healing for the skin. It will also soften callused areas on the skin.

Rosewater – Rose-scented water that is a byproduct of the production of rose essential oil. It is very softening, soothing, and toning to the skin. It can also be found as "rose hydrosol". Some rosewaters on the market have an alcohol base. Avoid using these, for the alcohol can dry your skin.

Rubbing Alcohol – A liquid that is poisonous when taken internally. It is used externally to extract herbal properties or to disperse essential oils. It has astringent and antibacterial properties.

Sea Salt – Salt that is evaporated from the sea or mined from former sea beds. It contains minerals and is used in baths to soften water and draw impurities from the body. Sea salt can be found available in larger coarse grains or finer ground pieces. The finely ground size dissolves more quickly in water for bath salt recipes.

Shea Butter – A semi-solid wax that comes from the seeds of the Karite tree which is found in Africa. It is very mild, softening, and moisturizing with a rich texture. It gives a smooth consistency to hand creams.

Sunflower Seeds – The seeds of the sunflower (*Helianthus* spp.) are used finely ground in masks and facial scrubs. Buy unsalted raw sunflower seeds. Store the seeds in the freezer or refrigerator as they have a tendency to become rancid quickly.

Super Silk – A liquid product that comes from the silk of the silkworm's spent cocoons. It contains amino acids and silk proteins that are able to penetrate the hair shaft giving it strength and the ability to hold moisture. It can also make your skin feel smooth. Use it in hair and skin care products.

Sweet Almond Oil – A clear pale yellow oil from almonds that is absorbed easily by the skin. It is recommended for all skin types and may be used full strength.

Table Salt – Use the non-iodized variety in tooth care preparations.

Tincture of Benzoin – A resin from the tree *Styrax benzoin* found in Asia, it is commonly found in an alcohol based tincture. It can be used as a preservative in mixtures. It is also protective and deodorizing to the skin. Do not use internally.

Turkey Red Oil – An oil, usually castor oil, that has been specially treated to make it dispersible in water. It is used in baths to soften the skin.

Vegetable Glycerin(e) – A sweet syrupy substance that is a humectant. It is used as an additive in body care products. Dilute with other ingredients—when used full strength it can pull moisture out of your skin.

Vinegar – A sour liquid obtained by acid fermentation of dilute alcohol fluids from a variety of sources. Softens and cleanses the skin and assists in maintaining the skin's acid mantle. Gives shine to hair when used as an after shampoo rinse. Apple cider vinegar is the most commonly used type of vinegar for skin and hair care.

Vitamin E – An antioxidant used in skin care products as a preservative. It comes measured in International Units, or IU. It is commonly available in gelcaps that can be punctured with a clean needle and the gelcap then squeezed to obtain the liquid. When shopping for Vitamin E, look for forms concentrated no less than 400 IU per gelcap. Less concentrated forms may interfere with the consistency of the body care product that you are making. Vitamin E can occasionally be found in a concentrated liquid form that may be measured then used as directed. Read the labels of Vitamin E bottles carefully before buying, and avoid those containing adulterants and/or synthetics. Look for the word "d-alpha tocopherol" on the label to assure that you are buying the correct product.

Wheat Germ Oil – A dark golden oil that contains Vitamins A, D, and E. It has a distinctive odor and heavy feel. Recommended for most skin types, but do not use it if you are allergic to wheat products. Use as an ingredient in skin preparations.

Witch Hazel – A distilled fluid of the bark from the shrub *Hamamelis virginiana* usually found in an alcohol base, it is astringent and anti-inflammatory. Do not use internally.

PATCH TEST FOR
SENSITIVITY CONCERNS

There is no guarantee that any specific ingredient will not cause an adverse reaction to your skin. Put a small dab of any substance or preparation that you have concerns about on the inside of your forearm, and put a Band-Aid over the spot. Leave the Band-Aid on overnight – if there is no redness or other signs of irritation the next day, the substance should be safe to use.

Herbs

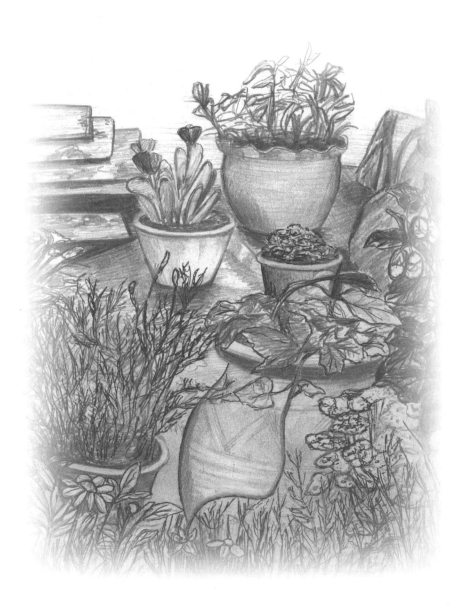

A number of years ago, a good friend of mine gave me some herb plants, divisions of existing plantings in her own gardens. The little knowledge that I had about herbs consisted of using them as seasoning for food from containers purchased at the store. I bought a reference book to learn more, and discovered that herbs were old standbys for many modern day products and, in many cases, have long since been replaced by synthetic substances. One of the many uses of herbs has been for making cosmetic preparations for the skin and body. I became intrigued with this idea, and kept reading, studying, and experimenting. The more I learned, the more intrigued I became with these plants' many uses. The number of herb plants in my gardens has increased several fold. The original six plants that my friend gave me have multiplied, and I have purchased and grown more varieties of herbs since. My reading and studying continues, and the uses of these plants have multiplied for me in numerous ways.

STARTING AN HERB GARDEN

Gardening is an activity that is very popular. It is a pastime that is relaxing mentally and emotionally. It can also provide a great means of physical exercise. Growing herbs is just a small segment of gardening, but it has become a major interest for veteran and novice gardeners alike.

Look for herb plants and seeds at your local garden center or nursery. Most seed and plant catalogues have a variety of herbs available as well.

There are many sources of information on herb gardening available. Look for local classes that feature herb gardening through your local library or nursery. The agricultural extension office in your state might also have information on growing herbs. Of course, look to the wide variety of books available on the subject. Seek these out in your local library. The Internet has informational websites on the topic as well. (Some fine books on herb gardening are listed in the Bibliography section of this book.)

Herbs are plants that are considered useful to man in any number of ways. Depending on the plant, uses include culinary, decorative, aromatic, cosmetic, and/or medicinal. The therapeutic value of herbs isn't just limited to topical or internal uses. Working with these plants in your garden – cultivating, harvesting, and enjoying them – is therapy in and of itself. Their fragrance teases you when you are pulling weeds from them, for any touch of the plants releases essential oils captured in the different plant parts. It even makes weeding a pleasant aromatic chore!

Growing and tending herbs gives you a personal connection with the plants that you are using. You get to know the different plants and find that you are drawn to certain ones for your own personal use. These tend to be the herbs that you use the most for various applications.

It is ideal to be able to grow, use, and harvest your own herbs. Whether you grow them yourself, harvest from the wild, or purchase fresh herbs, you must make absolutely sure that you are correctly identifying the plant. I recommend herb reference books that have photographs in them for positive identification. One of my favorites is *Rodale's Illustrated Encyclopedia of Herbs.* (See the Bibliography section for more information on herb reference books.)

COMMON NAME CAUTION

The common names of herbs can vary widely by region, with a common name in one part of the country meaning an entirely different plant than one with an identical common name in another part of the country. For this reason, I recommend that you familiarize yourself with the Latin binomial names of herb plants and refer to them when seeking out the herbs that you desire. These two-part scientific names give you first the genus name of the plant followed by the species name. A genus is a group of one or more plants that share a wide range of characteristics, and the species denotes a group of plants that are able to breed together to produce offspring that resemble themselves. Most reference books will give Latin binomial names of plants to help you with positive identification.

There are several ways to help you find herbs that are best suited for you. Seek out someone who is well versed in herbs and their uses and ask questions. Attend a class on herbs, or go to a local herb farm or nursery. Visit public gardens that feature herbs in their plantings. Read as much as you can on the subject. The popularity of herbs and their uses has made a wide variety of literature available on the topic. The more books and magazines about herbs that you read, the better informed you will become.

A word of caution – there can be potential drawbacks to using herbs. Just because herbs are "natural" doesn't necessarily mean that they are harmless. There can be limitations to using herbs, including the risk of allergies and sensitivities. Don't go overboard with your use of herbs or any other natural product. Seek out the advice of a health care professional for any abnormal physical conditions that you may have. Use moderation in your experimentation. Expand your knowledge base gradually and continually by reading and through other avenues of learning.

I have included the use of several herbs in the recipes in this book. Many are used in the form of essential oils, which will be covered in a later section. The herbs that I have used in their pure state are listed here with a brief explanation of each as it is used in this book.

WHAT'S IN A NAME?

If the word officinalis *is included in a plant's Latin binomial you can be relatively certain that the plant once was used medicinally. Check an updated herbal medicine source to validate the continued medicinal use of any given herb.*

Basil *(Ocimum basilicum)* – This herb has restorative, warming, and antibacterial effects for the skin. It can be used for facial and hair care. Use the leaves.

Calendula *(Calendula officinalis)* – This is a very beneficial herb for skin care with anti-inflammatory, antibacterial, and antifungal properties. It is beneficial for skin and hair care. Use the flower petals.

Catnip *(Nepeta cataria)* – Although this herb acts as a narcotic for our feline friends, it has the effect of relaxing humans. The pleasant aroma of this herb can help lull you to sleep when used as an ingredient in sleep pillows. The leaves of the plant are used.

Cinnamon *(Cinnamomum verum, C. zeylanicum)* – The ground form of the bark of this plant is used in mouthwashes for its ability to freshen and to stimulate gum circulation.

Clove *(Syzygium aromaticum, Eugenia carophyllata)* – The dried flower buds of this plant are used ground up and put into preparations for mouth care. Its strongly antiseptic properties help to freshen breath and stimulate gum circulation.

Dill *(Anethum graveolens)* – The seeds of this plant can be used for breath freshening.

Fennel *(Foeniculum vulgare)* – The seeds of this plant are aromatic and anti-inflammatory. An infusion of the seeds is cleansing and beneficial for aging skin. The somewhat sweet, licorice-flavored seeds can also be used for breath freshening.

German Chamomile *(Matricaria recutita)* – The fruity scented flowers of this plant are used in infusions for hair and skin care, and to help soothe tired, irritated eyes. It is a versatile plant—no wonder Peter Rabbit's mother gave him chamomile tea to calm him down after his difficult day with Mr. McGregor! If you suffer from ragweed allergy, German chamomile can potentially cause an adverse reaction with prolonged use.

Hops *(Humulus lupulus)* – Commonly known as an herb for flavoring beer, hops have sedative properties that help to promote sleep. In this book they are used as an ingredient in sleep pillows.

Lady's Mantle *(Alchemilla vulgaris)* – This striking looking plant has beautiful fluted leaves that contain an astringent property. It is used in infusions for facial care.

Lavender *(Lavandula angustifolia, L. officinalis)* – This herb, once considered old fashioned, has made an aromatic comeback. It can stimulate circulation and cleanse the skin. The aroma is considered to be relaxing. Its versatility makes it an ideal ingredient in skin and hair care products as well as a relaxing ingredient in sleep pillows. The flower buds of lavender are the most common part used and are widely available.

Lemon Balm *(Melissa officinalis)* – The lemon scented leaves of this herb have antibacterial properties that makes it a good choice when used in rinses for troubled skin conditions. The relaxing scent of the leaves can be a useful addition in sleep pillows.

Lemon Verbena *(Aloysia triphylla)* – This, the most lemon scented of all the "lemony" herbs, is astringent and aromatic. It can be used in facial care, and as an aromatic addition to sleep pillows. Use the leaves.

Mint *(Mentha* spp.) – Mints come in literally thousands of scents. Its mildly antiseptic properties are helpful for mouth and body care. In recipes calling for it, choose a mint that has a scent that pleases you. Use the leaves.

Parsley *(Petroselinum crispum)* – The leaves of this familiar culinary herb have a high chlorophyll content, making it an ideal breath freshener. It is also a nourishing addition to facial care products.

Rosemary *(Rosmarinus officinalis)* – An herb with many benefits, rosemary leaves stimulate the skin, lend strength to hair, and have deodorizing and antibacterial properties. It can be used widely in many skin and hair care products.

Sage *(Salvia officinalis)* – The leaves of this herb have astringent, antiseptic, and anti-inflammatory properties that make it useful for skin and mouth care. It can also be used as an ingredient in hair care.

Thyme *(Thymus vulgaris)* – Warming, antiseptic, antibacterial, antifungal, and astringent properties make this herb an appropriate addition to deodorants, facial and body care, and sleep pillows. Use the leaves.

Yarrow *(Achillea millifolium)* – Use the white flowered variety of this herb that is widely found in the wild. It has astringent and anti-inflammatory properties and can be used in skin care. Use the leaves and flowers.

STORING DRIED HERBS

Heat and light will cause a loss of effectiveness of dried herbs by allowing the plants' essential oils to evaporate. Preferably store dried herbs in glass containers and place the containers away from a direct source of heat and sunlight. Do not purchase dried herbs from any shop that exposes them to bright sunlight and/or a direct heat source, for their active properties will be diminished.

Essential Oils

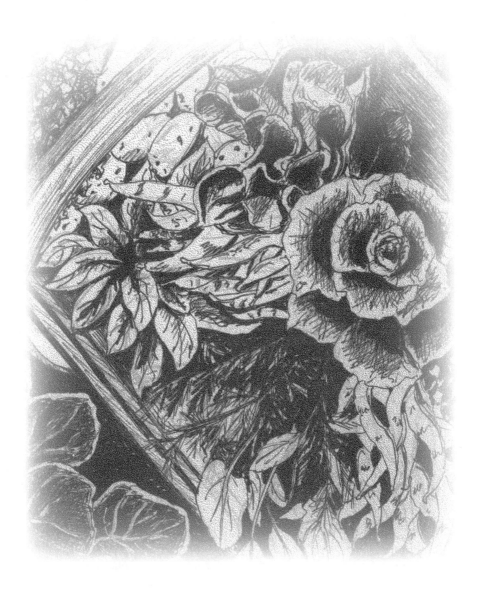

Essential oils are aromatic liquids derived from various parts of different herbs. Depending on the plant, essential oils are located in the bark, leaves, flowers, roots, seeds, or fruit. For example, the essential oils of orange, petitgrain, and neroli all come from various parts of citrus trees. Orange essential oil comes from the rind of the fruit, petitgrain comes from the leaves and twigs of the orange tree, and neroli comes from the orange blossoms.

There are different methods of extraction for essential oils depending on the plant parts from which the individual oils are derived. Expression or pressure extraction squeezes essential oils from appropriate plant parts. This is generally used for citrus essential oils such as lemon and orange. Steam distillation isolates volatile and water soluble parts of the plant and is used for lavender, myrrh, and sandalwood essential oils, among others. This steam distillation process is the method from which the majority of essential oils are extracted.

Although essential oils are usually liquid, a few are solid or semi-solid and must be further dissolved in a solvent such as alcohol, then the solvent removed in an evaporation process. Rose and jasmine essential oils are examples of the end product of this process. The word "absolute" after the name of the essential oil will tip you off that the solvent process has been used to obtain the essential oil.

A fairly new process called carbon dioxide extraction can be used to obtain essential oils thus eliminating the process of using solvents. The essential oils obtained from this process are quite expensive.

There are many chemical constituents in each essential oil that give each one its therapeutic properties. Please refer to the Bibliography section of this book for aromatherapy books for a further explanation.

Essential oils are typically very concentrated and are only used in measures of drops. They are used primarily through inhalation of the aroma and/or absorption through the skin. For safe topical use, essential oils must be diluted with another substance. As a general rule, essential oils are not meant to be taken internally. Absolutely do not take any essential oils internally without the supervision of a trained professional.

It takes different amounts of plant material to extract equal amounts of essential oil from different plants. For example, it takes sixty thousand rose petals to produce one ounce of pure essential oil of rose, making the end product a rather costly purchase. In contrast, it takes 220 pounds of lavender to make 7 pounds of essential oil, making its price much less than that of the rose.

Do not let the prices of essential oils discourage you from buying them. There are approximately 120 drops in ⅛ ounce of any essential oil. That gives you plenty for many different recipes. If the cost of certain essential oils seems prohibitive to you, find someone to split the cost and share the essential oil. There are certain shops that will also sell essential oils by the drop or in amounts even smaller than ⅛ of an ounce. Look around in your area or check the Internet for these sources. Check the Resources section of this book for possible sources of essential oils as well.

If stored in a dark glass container away from direct heat and light, the shelf life of essential oil is about two years. After that period of time, it can be used for fragrance but may lose therapeutic properties.

Feelings about different aromas vary from person to person. Scents that evoke positive feelings in some people may be repulsive to others. There is such a variety of essential oils that customizing a blend that appeals to you is relatively simple when you have some working knowledge of them.

HOW TO TELL THE REAL THING

Beware of essential oils that have been diluted or adulterated with other substances before purchase. The signs of adulteration are outlined here. Should any essential oil that you purchase have any of the following characteristics, then it should be assumed that it is not pure.

§ *Oily feel*

§ *Cool feel similar to that of rubbing alcohol (Peppermint essential oil is the exception to this rule. It evaporates quickly, producing a cool feeling on the skin.)*

> *When added to water, a milky color appears. Essential oils will float when added to water, and not mix with the water.*

> *Look for different prices for each individual essential oil when shopping. Bottles of different types of oil that have identical prices are probably either adulterated essential oils or synthetic fragrance oil.*

All of the recipes in this book are meant to use essential oils rather than synthetic fragrance oils. Essential oils have the reputation of being beneficial to your skin due to the therapeutic properties found in the plants from which they are obtained. Fragrance oils may smell good, but will not provide any therapeutic properties. Fragrance oils may also contain synthetic ingredients that can cause sensitivity reactions in some people.

CAUTIONS FOR USE

Essential oils are quite concentrated and should not be used carelessly. The following are some precautions to take when using essential oils.

> *Dilute essential oils prior to applying them to your skin. They may be diluted with carrier oils such as almond, olive, jojoba, or avocado. They may also be diluted in alcohol, powder, and soap mixtures.*

> *Mix essential oils thoroughly with other ingredients—contact with any "pockets" of undiluted oils can potentially cause irritation.*

> *Do not use essential oils around your eyes. The fumes from the evaporating oils can be extremely irritating to them, causing redness and tearing.*

> *Use care when using essential oils on babies and children, pregnant women, nursing mothers, persons with certain physical conditions, and the elderly. Each of these groups have special precautions when it comes to using essential oils. Consult a reliable aromatherapy book for guidelines on using essential oils in any of these special circumstances (See the Bibliography section of this book for some choices.)*

§ *Do not use more than recommended amounts of any essential oil in a given recipe. Increasing the amount of essential oil can increase the likelihood of adverse reactions.*

§ *Essential oils are quite volatile, which means they evaporate readily. To avoid losing the oils before you can enjoy their benefits, do not add to hot or very warm mixtures.*

§ *Essential oils are flammable—do not let any essential oil come in direct contact with a direct heat source or open flame.*

§ *Measure essential oils by the drop. To measure, use a clean dry eye dropper or use the built-in dropper that comes in many essential oil bottles.*

ESSENTIAL OIL PRECAUTIONS FOR PREGNANT WOMEN

This is a partial list of essential oils for pregnant women to avoid. Consult an aromatherapy book or aromatherapist for further information.

basil	fennel	pennyroyal
carrot seed	frankincense	peppermint
camphor	hyssop	rose
cedarwood	juniper	rosemary
cinnamon	marjoram	sage
clary sage	myrrh	thyme
clove	oregano	verbena

Here is the list of the essential oils used in recipes in this book. To substitute one essential oil for another one in the recipes, use this list as a guide or refer to an aromatherapy book (See the Bibliography section for some book choices.). The properties for each essential oil are listed in parentheses.

Basil (*Ocimum basilicum*) – It has a spicy aroma. It may be used in skin care products for oily or normal skin types. (cleansing, circulatory stimulant, antiseptic, and toning)

Bergamot (*Citrus bergamia*) – Use for normal, troubled, or oily skin and hair. It has a lovely aroma. (deodorizing and astringent)

Carrot Seed (*Daucas carota*) – Protects aged and wrinkled skin. Rejuvenates and helps to heal irritated, dry, and chapped skin conditions. (antioxidant)

Cedarwood (also known as **Atlas Cedarwood**) (*Cedrus atlantica*) –This essential oil is stimulating to the skin's circulation. It is also soothing to troubled skin. The woodsy aroma seems masculine to me. It would be a good addition to a toner or aftershave for men. (antiseptic, antifungal, circulatory stimulant, and astringent)

Cinnamon (*Cinnamomum zeylanicum, C. verum*) – The cinnamon leaf essential oil is less irritating than cinnamon bark oil, which is not recommended for body care. Its fresh spicy aroma and astringent and antiseptic properties are good for mouth care or skin care. Use sparingly. (astringent and antiseptic)

Clary Sage (*Salvia sclarea*) – This one is appropriate when used on troubled or wrinkled skin. It is also deodorizing. Do not confuse this essential oil with sage (*Salvia officinalis*) oil, which has a greater potential for harmful side effects. The use of clary sage essential oil is not recommended if you have had any alcohol intake because it is reported to cause nightmares and potentiate the effects of alcohol. (relaxant, antiseptic, and deodorizing)

Clove (*Eugenia caryophyllata, Syzygium aromaticum*) – A spicy smelling essential oil that is good for softening calluses and for foot care. It can also be used in mouth care products. Use sparingly – in large amounts it can be quite irritating to tissues. (antifungal)

Cypress (*Cupressus sempervirens*) – This essential oil is useful in skin care, especially when one is troubled with fragile or broken capillaries. It is deodorizing and great for use in foot care as well. (antiseptic, astringent, and deodorizing)

Eucalyptus (*Eucalyptus globulus, E. radiata, E. smithii*) – The aroma of this essential oil is easily recognizable as an ingredient in products for cold care. It can be put to good use on oily or irritated skin. (deodorizing, antiseptic, antifungal, and antibacterial)

Frankincense (also known as **Olibanum**) (*Boswellia carteri*) – This essential oil is a real workhorse when it comes to skin care. It helps prevent wrinkles by strengthening connective tissue. It will help to soften and heal aging, oily, and/or irritated skin. (antiseptic, anti-inflammatory, emollient, astringent, and cell regenerative)

Geranium (also known as **Rose Geranium**) (*Pelargonium graveolens*) – This essential oil can be used for all skin types. It can help to smooth lines and wrinkles on aged skin. The scent of rose geranium essential oil is similar to that of rose essential oil, and can be used as a substitute for the scent, but do not expect it to replace the active properties of rose essential oil. (cleansing, anti-inflammatory, and antiseptic)

German Chamomile (*Matricaria recutita*) – This essential oil has a deep blue color due to components called azulenes. It is appropriately used on troubled, irritated, and/or sensitive skin. (antibacterial, anti-inflammatory, and soothing)

Ginger (*Zingiber officinalis*) – This essential oil is warmly aromatic. It can be used to enhance the effects of a foot soak. Due to its potentially irritating effect on the skin, use only in small amounts in weak dilution. (antiseptic, anti-inflammatory, and circulatory stimulant)

Grapefruit (*Citrus paradisii*) – Oily skin will benefit from this essential oil. It is also an appropriate addition to deodorants, lip balms, and skin toners. (antiseptic, deodorizing, and cleansing)

Jasmine (*Jasminum grandiflorum, J. officinale*) – A rich luxurious smelling essential oil that adds a heady floral scent to baths and skin care products. Its high price leads me to use it sparingly, making it all the more special when I use it. (emollient, astringent, moisturizing, and soothing)

Juniper (*Juniperus communis*) – The clean aroma of this essential oil makes it a good addition to deodorants. It is also helpful for oily, irritated, or congested skin. It makes a helpful addition to products for normal or oily hair. Avoid using juniper essential oil if you have any kidney problems or a history of them. (cleansing, toning, astringent, antiseptic, and circulatory stimulant)

Lavender (*Lavandula officinalis, L. angustifolia*) – Versatile is the word that best describes lavender essential oil. It can be used in products for the hair or skin and is good for any skin type. It is particularly useful when used on chapped skin, sunburn, or wrinkled skin. (cell regenerative, toning, anti-inflammatory, antiseptic, and deodorizing)

PHOTOTOXICITY AND CITRUS DERIVED ESSENTIAL OILS

Certain essential oils can cause adverse reactions to the skin when applied and then exposed to sunlight or the rays from a tanning booth. Adverse reactions can include the burning and blistering of the skin and/or abnormal darkening of the skin. The darkening effect can last for several months. Individuals who have a history of skin cancers, moles, and abnormal pigmentations can be more susceptible to reactions. Avoid direct sun or tanning booth exposure for 6 hours after topical application of any of these essential oils. Essential oils that are derived from citrus sources are the main culprits of phototoxicity reactions. They include:

Bergamot	*Lemon*	*Mandarin or Tangerine*
Grapefruit	*Lime*	*Orange*

Lemon (*Citrus limonum, C. limon*) – Recommended for all skin types, this essential oil is as fragrant as the sunny yellow fruit from which it is derived! It can be used in lip care, skin care, nail care, and hair care. It can reduce puffiness and wrinkles in the skin. It will add shine to the hair. (antiseptic, astringent, and toning)

Lime (*Citrus aurantifolia*) – A refreshingly fragrant essential oil that will lend an uplifting aroma to baths and skin care. (astringent)

Myrrh (also known as **Opopanax**) *(Commiphora myrrha)* – This essential oil is particularly effective when used in mouth and gum care. It can also lend help to skin that is sensitive, chapped, irritated, or wrinkled. (astringent, antiseptic, and antifungal)

Neroli *(Citrus aurantium)* – A fragrant, exotic smelling oil that is derived from orange blossoms, neroli essential oil is a lovely addition to skin care products. It is also appropriately used in the bath. (antiseptic and deodorizing)

Orange (also known as **Sweet Orange**) *(Citrus sinensis)* – The sweet and fresh smelling aroma of this essential oil often reminds me of the orange candy suckers that we ate as children. It can be used on a variety of skin types in products for the skin and bath. (toning and circulatory stimulant)

Palmarosa *(Cymbopogon martini)* – Derived from a grass that is native to Central and South America, palmarosa essential oil can lend a healing touch to skin care products. (antiseptic and antibacterial)

Patchouli *(Pogostemon patchouli, P. cablin)* – Those of you old enough to remember will recall patchouli oil being used, sometimes to excess, in the 1960's. Then and now you either loved or hated the aroma. I am personally in the "love it" category for patchouli essential oil. Its rich, woodsy fragrance lends a healing touch to skin care products and deodorants. It can also lend balance to oil and moisture levels in the skin. (deodorizing, anti-inflammatory, antiseptic, and cell regenerative)

Peppermint *(Mentha piperita)* – This essential oil smells like Christmas candy. It is helpful to oily, irritated, and/or congested skin. Peppermint essential oil evaporates quickly, lending a cool feeling to skin care products. (antiseptic, anti-inflammatory, astringent, and toning)

Pine *(Pinus sylvestris)* – A rejuvenating fragrance, pine essential oil is a good addition to bath products. (antiseptic, deodorizing, stimulating, and toning)

Rose *(Rosa damascena)* – One of the more expensive essential oils, the scent of roses makes this worth the cost. It can be used in skin care and bath products. It is helpful for wrinkled and chapped skin. There are a couple of forms of rose essential oil available. Rose otto is steam distilled. Rose concrete or absolute is solvent extracted. (antiseptic, astringent, and toning)

Rosemary *(Rosmarinus officinalis)* – This essential oil comes from my most favorite herb. It is best used in products for oily or normal hair and skin. It has a reputation for aiding in strengthening hair. (astringent, antiseptic, deodorizing, circulatory stimulant, and cell regenerative)

Rosewood (also known as ***Bois de Rose***) *(Aniba rosaeodora)* – This essential oil can be used on normal or wrinkled skin. The scent seems some-what masculine to me, and could be used in aftershave or skin toning preparations for men. (deodorizing, antiseptic, cell regenerative, toning, and revitalizing)

Sandalwood *(Santalum album)* – A strong exotic scent that is healing for chapped, irritated, and/or dry skin conditions. Its properties can help to maintain the skin's elasticity. (antiseptic, emollient, cell regenera-tive, and soothing)

Tangerine (also known as **Mandarin**) *(Citrus reticulata)* – Another one of the clean fresh-smelling citrus essential oils, tangerine can be used in skin or lip care products. (antiseptic and toning)

Tea Tree *(Melaleuca alternifolia)* – Often called a medicine chest in a bottle, tea tree essential oil can aid in healing troubled or chapped skin. (antibacterial, antifungal, antiseptic, and anti-inflammatory)

Thyme *(Thymus vulgaris)* – As soon as you smell this essential oil, you will recognize it as an ingredient of a popular medicinal-type mouthwash. It can be used on troubled skin and in deodorants. Do not use if you have a history of thyroid or seizure problems. (antiseptic, circulatory stimulant, and toning)

Ylang ylang *(Cananga odorata)* – The peculiar sounding name of this es-sential oil means "flower of flowers". It has a rich sweet floral scent. It can be used in skin care products for normal, oily, dry, aged and /or mature skin types. (emollient and antiseptic)

Improving Your Appearance Naturally

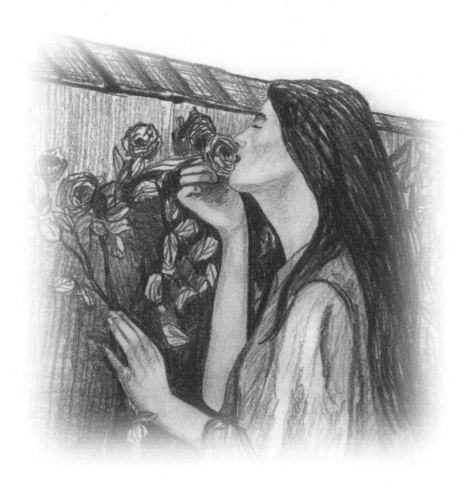

*W*hen it comes right down to it, there are no magic potions, treatments, or ingredients that will improve your appearance instantly. Different cosmetics do help to protect and care for your body's appearance, but before you reach for any products or ingredients to make some products, investigate some other ways to take care of your appearance. Here are some simple steps to take that will help to ensure a healthy attractive appearance.

Accept the Unchangeable

Most of us don't look like high fashion models, nor will we ever look like them. Some aspects of your appearance that you don't like are yours for life, and you can't do anything about them. Learn to accept your given appearance and maximize your strengths. We are all individuals and should enjoy and celebrate our differences. Remember that any appearance that reflects radiant health is beautiful.

Rest and Sleep

First of all, a good night's sleep is essential for a healthy appearance. It is always obvious when you look at a person whether or not they have slept well. Avoid medications for getting to sleep—a healthy, natural sleep is much better for you. Do not drink anything containing caffeine during the second half of your day. Caffeine is a stimulant and can interfere with your attempts to go to sleep. Try to use fragrance contained in a sleep pillow to help you to relax. Keep your mind free from that list in your head of things to do tomorrow and forget the conflicts at work that you have to address in the morning. If you don't, these situations will rerun over and over in your head when you close your eyes and help to keep you awake. To clear your mind, take some slow deep breaths and visualize a calm soothing picture in your mind that will help to relax you as you are lying in bed.

Even the pillow that you choose to sleep on will aid in improving your appearance. Pick the softest pillow that you can find. It is kinder to the delicate skin on your face, avoiding pushing and stretching the skin which can encourage the formation of wrinkles.

Washing and Cleansing

The way that you use water externally has a big effect on your appearance. Washing your skin too often can have negative effects regardless of the type of skin that you have. Too much washing of oily skin can stimulate the oil glands to produce more, making oily skin oilier, while frequent washing of dry skin makes it drier by washing away any oil that is present on the skin. Taking a bath or shower once a day should be adequate for you unless you are engaged in an activity that causes you to get extra dirty and sweaty. The act of bathing for longer than 20 minutes can be tiring to your body. Baths and showers that are too warm can dry out your skin and drain your energy. Water that is a warm or lukewarm temperature is ideal.

At the most, washing your face twice a day should be enough. It is acceptable to use soap on any type of skin. Soap is alkaline and does alter the skin's acid mantle briefly, but the skin's sebum will help to readjust the acid mantle to its normal level. If you have dry skin, try to avoid harsh deodorant soaps. Dry or sensitive skin types should use milder types of soap with minimal amounts of chemical additives. Use a small amount of soap and rinse every trace of it from your skin, patting, not rubbing, it dry. The use of lukewarm water for cleaning is preferable to very hot water.

Washing your hands is, of course, a frequent and necessary activity during the course of a day. Use soap and water for maximum cleaning of your hands. Rub your hands together briskly while washing them. The friction created by rubbing helps to remove soil and any undesirable bacteria that may be present. Dry your hands thoroughly and apply cream or lotion as needed to prevent your hands from drying out and to help maintain the skin's integrity. To further protect your hands, wear gloves when doing any task that is potentially damaging to your skin.

Intact skin is your body's first line of defense against the introduction of bacteria that can cause infections or other undesirable substances that can be potentially irritating and cause problems. Use moisturizers to help keep your skin soft and supple. Avoid substances or external conditions that will dry and/or irritate your skin, making it more prone to breakdown.

Other Facial Cleansing

I strongly discourage you from using facial steams or facial saunas. These procedures expose your skin to a concentrated amount of very hot moisture which can be potentially damaging to the delicate skin on your face. Facial steam is absolutely contraindicated on facial skin that is acne prone, very dry, or prone to broken or fragile capillaries. Another danger of exposing the face to hot steam is the potential for burns. As an alternative to steam, use soft cloths soaked in warm water or herbal infusion, applying them to your face for about 15 minutes. This will open your skin's pores for cleansing purposes. Follow cleansing with an application of toner or astringent. This alternative to facial steams should not be used more than every two to three days for oily skin types, and weekly or every other week for other skin types.

Humidity

The amount of humidity in your home is an important factor in maintaining the moisture levels in your skin and mucous membranes. Dry air can draw moisture out your skin and mucous membranes, making both feel tight and uncomfortable. This can be a problem especially in the fall and winter months. A simple table top humidifier will greatly improve the moisture content of the air in your home. Even bowls of water placed near heat registers will help to increase the humidity. Add a few drops of essential oil to the water for a pleasing scent.

Getting Enough Fluid Inside

You cannot keep your skin well hydrated without drinking enough fluids. All the creams and moisturizers in the world won't keep your skin moist if you don't hydrate from the inside. Drink six to eight 8-ounce glasses of fluid a day, more if you are perspiring heavily. Water is the fluid of choice for keeping hydrated, although other beverages can be drunk as well. Drink beverages with caffeine in moderation. Caffeine is a diuretic, causing you to excrete more fluids. Don't think that you aren't losing water if you lead a sedentary lifestyle, for you lose moisture while breathing in and out and even the most sedentary person perspires.

Persons with heart problems, kidney disorders, or those taking certain medications should be cautious about the amount of their daily fluid intake. If you suffer from any illness or abnormal physical condition, consult your health care professional about how much fluid intake is appropriate for you.

Diet and Nutrition

A proper diet is important to your health and well-being, including the condition of your skin. Eat lots of fresh fruits and vegetables, preferably organically grown if you can find them. Keep fat intake to the recommended 30% or lower of your daily intake. When adding carbohydrates to your diet, stick to the least refined products available to you. Refined carbohydrates have had all of the nutrients and fiber removed to make the product look nice and white, then the nutrients are artificially put back into the product. This makes no sense to me when all of the nutrients and fiber were there in the first place. There are many books and publications available on nutrition and a healthy diet. Read them and stay informed.

Your Skin and the Sun

Too much sun exposure is a notorious cause of skin problems. Sun damage to the skin can promote wrinkles, give you sunburn, and make you susceptible to all forms of skin cancer. To avoid sunburn and other skin damage due to overexposure to the sun, wear sunscreen, wear a hat when outside, and avoid direct sun exposure at the peak times of the day between 10 AM and 2 PM. For goodness sake, don't use tanning booths! At the absolute best, you are giving your skin the opportunity to age prematurely. At the worst you are increasing the risk of doing irreversible harm to your skin and body. Avoid them!

Exercise

Get enough exercise. Recent research has shown that even 15 minute periods of exercise at a time are beneficial for you. Take a walk, ride a bicycle, play tag with your children! Get outside and do yard work or garden. Clean the house. You know what you need to do. Just get out there and do it.

Promote Internal Peace and Calm

Finally, take care of and take responsibility for your inner self. Resolve your inner tensions and deal with your conflicts. Find humor in your life—laughter is a great tension reliever. Find an interest or passion and get involved in it. Relax and take some time out for yourself daily, even if it is only 15 minutes of your day. If you are bogged down with a lot of negative emotions and they are not being dealt with, it shows in your appearance. Turn to professional guidance if you feel totally overwhelmed. Emphasizing the positives in your life and achieving some form of inner peace will reward you with a better outlook and, consequently, a better appearance.

Try some of the above ways to help you feel and look your best. If you feel healthy, you will look healthy. None of these tips will make you beautiful overnight. It takes some effort and time to achieve an appearance of health and well-being. Use common sense and work to improve your daily life. Ultimately you will see results that will please you – both inside and out.

Getting Started

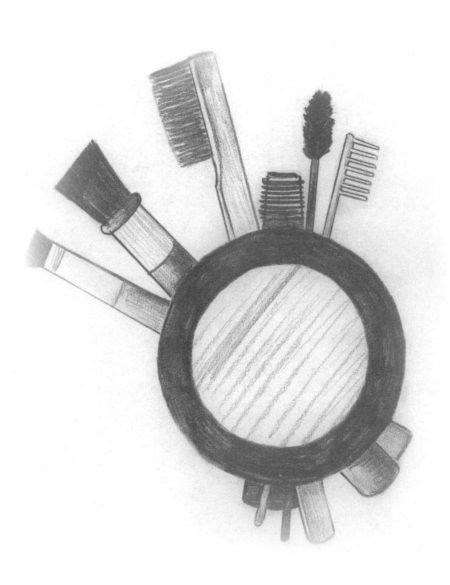

*A*t the beginning, make small batches of any of the body care products in this book. This will help you not to waste a large amount of ingredients if any of your recipes don't turn out the way you expected. Making small batches of a product will also decrease the chances of spoilage. Keep in mind that even with the addition of preservatives such as Vitamin E, grapefruit seed extract, and/or tincture of benzoin, the shelf life of these products is usually not as long as those of a commercially produced product.

SHELF LIFE OF HOMEMADE
BODY CARE PRODUCTS

There are some steps that you can take to extend the shelf life of your custom made products. They are outlined for you here.

§ *Make sure that all utensils used when making your products are scrupulously clean.*

§ *Store products in glass containers when possible. Amber or brown colored glass is preferable.*

§ *Store products away from heat sources and direct sunlight. Both of these factors increase the risk of spoilage and decrease the potency of the active ingredients in the product.*

§ *Products can be stored in the refrigerator to prolong shelf life.*

§ *Creams can be stored in the freezer for an even longer shelf life. Before using, remove them from the freezer and let them thaw at room temperature.*

§ *Herbal infusions can be stored in the refrigerator if there are leftovers, but they must be used within three days or discarded.*

§ *Should any product change color, develop mold, or develop an "off" odor or appearance, discard them immediately.*

§ *Be sure to add Vitamin E, grapefruit seed extract, or tincture of benzoin, if called for in the recipe. These are natural preservatives and will aid in keeping your products fresh.*

For uniform consistency, all products that have been melted when combined must be whisked occasionally while cooling to stay blended and prevent lumps. The addition of an emulsifier in the form of liquid lecithin will keep oil-based and water-based ingredients from separating out in the final product. Occasionally some separation of ingredients does occur in a finished product. Simply mix or shake the product before using should this occur.

OTHER POINTS TO CONSIDER

§ *Label all finished products with its ingredients.*

§ *Custom-made products such as creams and oils are more concentrated than their commercial counterparts. Use smaller amounts when applying them to your skin. A little goes a long way.*

Enjoy trying these recipes. Should you want to customize any of them, review the sections on ingredients, essential oils, and herbs, and experiment. Substitute any of the given oils, clay, essential oils, and herbs for a similar ingredient according to your preferences and needs. The possibilities of combinations are nearly endless. If you aren't feeling adventuresome or just don't want to experiment, stick with the recipes that I have provided for you. They have been tried both by myself and by others to make sure that they are useful and useable.

HELPFUL HINT FOR
CREATING PRODUCTS

Keep a pencil or pen and a piece of scrap paper handy when experimenting with combining ingredients to create your own recipes. Write down what and how much of each ingredient that you add. If you like the end result, you have a brand new recipe that is a "keeper" – and you have a record of it besides!

MEASUREMENT ABBREVIATIONS

Tbsp. = tablespoon   *tsp. = teaspoon*   *3 tsp. = 1 tablespoon*

Deodorant

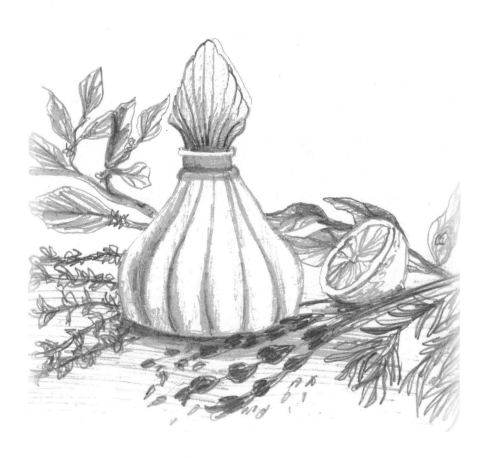

$\mathcal{U}$nderarm odor occurs when the by-products of perspiration break down when exposed to air and bacteria is formed. The following preparations contain ingredients with antibacterial and deodorizing properties. Before applying these deodorants, shake well. Use cotton pads to apply them to your skin in the underarm area or place in a spray bottle and spray on the skin. Let the application dry before getting dressed. Avoid using underarm deodorants immediately after shaving. Freshly shaved skin has a greater tendency to become irritated. Discontinue the use of any deodorant if redness, a rash, or other signs of irritation develop.

LEMON-LAVENDER DEODORANT

A fragrant combination of essential oils help to keep odors away!

Mix the following ingredients together:

1 Tbsp. pure grain alcohol
2 drops lemon essential oil
2 drops lavender essential oil
1 drop tea tree essential oil

After the above ingredients are thoroughly mixed, add:

1 Tbsp. witch hazel extract
10 drops grapefruit seed extract

Mix all ingredients together thoroughly. Store in a bottle with a lid or sprayer. Shake well before using.

LEMON-THYME DEODORANT

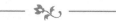

The serious bacteria-fighting power of tea tree and thyme essential oils combines with the refreshing scent of lemon.

 1 Tbsp. witch hazel extract
 1 Tbsp. rubbing alcohol
 2 drops tea tree essential oil
 2 drops thyme essential oil
 1 drop lemon essential oil

Mix the above ingredients thoroughly. Store in a bottle with a lid or sprayer. Shake well before using.

BERGAMOT-PATCHOULI DEODORANT

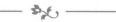

The addition of patchouli essential oil adds an exotic scent to this recipe. Note: The vinegar smell will not linger in this recipe once it is applied to the skin.

 1 Tbsp. apple cider vinegar
 1 Tbsp. witch hazel extract
 15 drops grapefruit seed extract
 3 drops bergamot essential oil
 3 drops patchouli essential oil

Mix the above ingredients together. Store in a bottle with a lid or sprayer. Shake well before using.

LEMON-PATCHOULI DEODORANT

When well-diluted, grapefruit seed extract makes a useful bacteria-fighting addition to deodorant preparations.

> **2 Tbsp. apple cider vinegar**
> **2 Tbsp. witch hazel extract**
> **10 drops grapefruit seed extract**
> **5 drops patchouli essential oil**
> **3 drops lemon essential oil**
> **2 drops myrrh essential oil**

Mix the above ingredients together thoroughly. Store in a bottle with a lid or sprayer. Shake well before using.

LAVENDAR-ROSEMARY DEODORANT

One of my favorites, rosemary essential oil combines with those of lavender and tea tree for effective deodorizing.

> **½ cup witch hazel extract**
> **25 drops grapefruit seed extract**
> **8 drops lavender essential oil**
> **5 drops tea tree essential oil**
> **3 drops rosemary essential oil**

Mix the above ingredients together thoroughly. Store in a bottle with a lid or sprayer. Shake well before using.

PEPPERMINT-JUNIPER DEODORANT

An herbal scent that imparts a cooling feel.

2 Tbsp. pure grain alcohol
3 drops peppermint essential oil
1 drop rosemary essential oil
1 drop juniper essential oil

Mix the above ingredients together thoroughly. Store in a bottle with a lid or sprayer. Shake well before using.

ROSEMARY-THYME DEODORANT

The herbal and lemon scent makes this combination a winner. Try it and see what you think!

2 Tbsp. apple cider vinegar
1 Tbsp. witch hazel extract
3 drops thyme essential oil
2 drops lemon essential oil
2 drops rosemary essential oil

Mix the above ingredients together thoroughly. Store in a bottle with a lid or sprayer. Shake well before using.

LAVENDER-PATCHOULI DEODORANT

This recipe combines three deodorizing essential oils.

½ cup rubbing alcohol
1 tsp. grapefruit seed extract
10 drops lavender essential oil
6 drops patchouli essential oil
4 drops tea tree essential oil

Mix the above ingredients together thoroughly. Store in a bottle with a lid or sprayer. Shake well before using.

DEODORIZING ESSENTIAL OILS

The following essential oils are considered to have deodorizing properties and can be most effectively used in deodorant mixtures.

bergamot	juniper	rosewood
clary sage	grapefruit	tangerine
cypress	neroli	tea tree
eucalyptus	patchouli	thyme
lavender	pine	
lemon	rosemary	

Eye Care

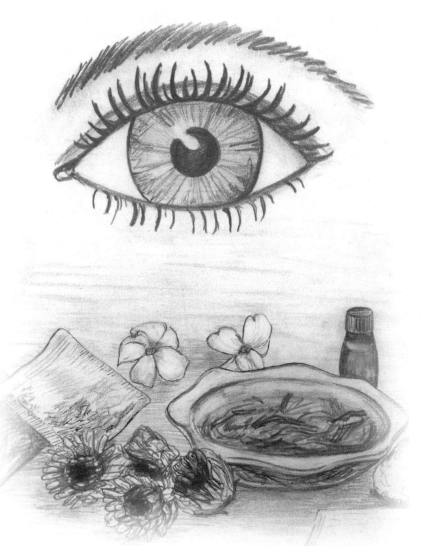

*Y*our eyes are very important to you and must be treated with the utmost of care. Pollutants in the atmosphere and/or a lack of sleep can cause redness and irritation that can easily be alleviated with some simple herbal treatments. There are several ingredients that can be used around your eyes. Recipes containing these ingredients are safe and gentle when used as directed.

The skin around the eyes requires extra care because it is more fragile than the skin on the rest of your face. It should not be rubbed or scrubbed hard, as this can stretch the skin too much and help to cause the formation of wrinkles and lines.

The simple act of getting enough sleep will go far to reduce redness and dark circles under the eyes. If you haven't been getting enough sleep, use one of the following Eye Soother recipes and close your eyes and rest for 15 minutes. You and your eyes will feel refreshed afterwards.

SPECIAL PRECAUTIONS REGARDING YOUR EYES

Refer to the following list if you are experiencing any unusual problems with your eyes.

- *Report eye redness that doesn't go away, itching or burning eyes, visual disturbances, and/or unusual drainage or discharge from the eyes to your health care professional.*

- *Do not introduce any drops or foreign substances into your eyes without professional supervision.*

- *Avoid putting concentrated substances such as essential oils around your eyes. These can cause burning, stinging, redness, and watering.*

- *Discard eye makeup after 3 months. Old makeup can be an ideal medium for bacterial growth, which can potentially cause an eye infection.*

- *Make eye care products in small quantities. It is better to make small quantities frequently than to make large quantities that will sit around indefinitely and become contaminated with bacteria.*

Avoid applying rich creams and oils around your eyes. They can promote puffiness and even cause possible allergic reactions.

CHAMOMILE EYE SOOTHER

Chamomile tea bags with rare exceptions contain German chamomile although they are not always labeled as such. If you have an allergy to ragweed, use of German chamomile on a regular basis may produce allergic reactions.

⅛ chamomile tea bags
1 cup distilled water

Heat the distilled water to boiling and remove from the heat after it comes to a full rolling boil. Add the tea bags to the water. Allow the water to cool to lukewarm with the tea bags in it. Remove the tea bags and squeeze the excess fluid from them. Place the tea bags on your closed eyes. Leave them in place for 15 minutes. Remove them from your eyes and discard. The infusion can be stored in the refrigerator for up to three days and used as a hair rinse or facial rinse.

CALENDULA EYE SOOTHER

2 Tbsp. dried calendula blossoms
⅓ cup distilled water

Add the calendula blossoms to the water and bring to a boil. Reduce the heat and simmer covered for about 10 minutes. Strain the blossoms from the infusion and allow the infusion to cool to room temperature. Soak gauze squares, clean cloth squares or cotton pads in the infusion, squeeze out the excess, and place on closed eyes. Leave the squares on your eyes for 15 minutes. Remove and discard. The leftover infusion can be stored in the refrigerator for up to three days and used as a skin or hair rinse.

FENNEL EYE SOOTHER

3 Tbsp. crushed fennel seeds
⅓ cup distilled water

Add the crushed seeds to the water and bring to a boil. Reduce the heat and simmer covered for about 15 minutes. Remove from heat and immediately strain the seeds from the infusion, and let the infusion cool to room temperature. Soak gauze squares, clean cloth squares, or cotton pads in the infusion, squeeze out the excess fluid, and place on closed eyes for 15 minutes. Remove and discard. The leftover infusion can be stored in the refrigerator for up to three days and used as a skin rinse.

TIRED EYE RELIEF

½ cup dried lavender buds
½ cup distilled water

Bring the distilled water to a boil. Pour over the lavender buds, cover, and let steep for 15 minutes. Strain the lavender buds from the infusion and discard. Let the infusion cool to room temperature. Soak gauze squares, clean cloth squares, or cotton pads in the infusion, squeeze out the excess fluid, and place on closed eyes for 15 minutes. Remove and discard. The leftover infusion can be stored in the refrigerator for up to three days and used as a skin rinse.

Natural Beauty Basics

AROUND THE EYE OIL

This formula is very light. It could also be used to remove eye makeup.

> 1/8 tsp. rosehip seed oil
> 10 drops evening primrose oil
> 10 drops Vitamin E (use 400 IU per gelcap or concentrated liquid
>   Vitamin E 32,000 IU per fluid ounce)
> 10 drops jojoba oil

Mix all of the ingredients together. Gently massage a drop or two of the mixture into the skin around your eyes. Store any remaining oil in a small glass bottle.

NOURISHING EYE OIL

> ½ tsp. jojoba oil
> 1 drop carrot seed essential oil
> 400 IU Vitamin E

Mix all of the ingredients together. Gently massage a drop or two of the mixture into the skin around your eyes. Store any remaining oil in a small glass bottle.

ROSY EYE MAKEUP REMOVER

Read the labels on your products. Make sure that you are purchasing a hydrosol. Do not use rosewater that contains alcohol for removing eye makeup. The alcohol can be very irritating to your eyes, causing redness and watering.

Rose hydrosol

Using soft cotton pads or cotton balls, saturate them with rose hydrosol and gently wipe away any eye makeup.

Variations: Substitute lavender hydrosol or neroli (orange blossom) hydrosol for the rose hydrosol, and use as directed.

CUSTOMIZED EYE MAKEUP REMOVER

lavender, German chamomile, OR calendula infused oil (See instructions for making infused oil in the Bath and Body Oil section of this book.)

Saturate soft cotton pads or cotton balls with the herbal infused oil, and gently wipe away any eye makeup.

Lip Care

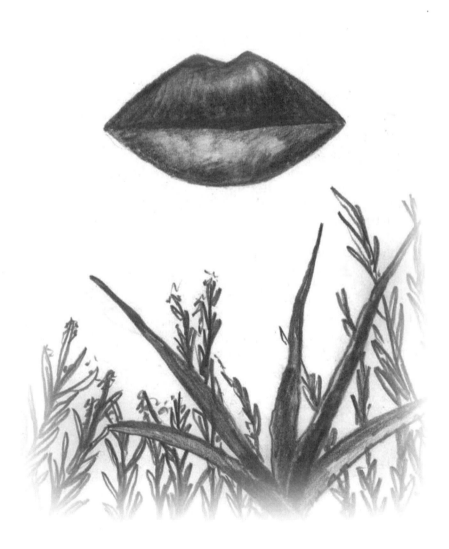

Commercial products for lip care are widely available, but are frequently full of artificial fragrances, flavors, and colors. The addition of artificial ingredients do not enhance the effectiveness of the product and could cause problems with people who have sensitivities to them. They also have to be reapplied frequently to maintain lip moisture. I have found that the following recipes do not require frequent applications. They have the ability to keep your lips soft and moist for longer periods of time.

CITRUS LIP GLOSS

When I sent a sample of this to my friend, she called to say, "This tastes good, send me more!" The citrus essential oils and honey combine to make this gloss a tasty product that will keep your lips soft and moist for some time.

> 3 Tbsp. sweet almond oil
> 2 tsp. beeswax (pearls or solid beeswax grated and measured)
> 1 tsp. aloe vera gel
> 1 tsp. honey
> 800 IU Vitamin E
> 4 drops lemon essential oil
> 3 drops tangerine essential oil

Melt the beeswax and sweet almond oil together in a heat proof container over boiling water. When the beeswax is melted, remove from the heat. Add the honey and Vitamin E, mixing briskly with a wire whisk. Add the aloe vera gel and stir into the mixture. Add the essential oils and stir in well. Pour into a low wide-mouth jar.

HEALING LIP GLOSS

This is a more "serious" lip gloss. It's not as tasty as the Citrus Lip Gloss, but has lots of protective and moisturizing qualities with the addition of the coconut oil and carrot seed essential oil. It also includes the healing properties of tea tree essential oil.

> 3 Tbsp. apricot kernel oil
> 2 tsp. beeswax (pearls or solid beeswax grated and measured)
> 1 tsp. coconut oil
> 800 IU Vitamin E
> 5 drops carrot seed essential oil
> 3 drops lemon essential oil
> 2 drops tea tree essential oil

Place the beeswax, apricot kernel oil, and coconut oil in a heat proof container and place over boiling water. When the mixture has melted, remove it from the heat. Add the Vitamin E, mixing with a wire whisk. Add the essential oils and mix well. Pour into a low wide-mouth jar.

EXTRA CARE FOR LIPS

This recipe is very protective, tastes good, and has a nice consistency. It is my hands-down favorite for lip care and many of my acquaintances agree.

> 1 Tbsp. beeswax (pearls or solid beeswax grated and measured)
> 1 Tbsp. avocado oil
> 1 tsp. vegetable glycerine
> ½ tsp. honey
> ⅛ tsp. liquid lecithin
> 6 drops grapefruit, orange OR lemon essential oil
> 4 drops tea tree essential oil

In a separate container, mix the honey and vegetable glycerine and set aside. Place the beeswax and avocado oil in a heat proof container and place over boiling water. When the mixture has melted, remove it from the heat. To the melted beeswax and oil mixture add Vitamin E and liquid lecithin. Slowly add the honey and vegetable glycerine mixture, stirring constantly. This will solidify rather quickly. Add the essential oils and mix well. Store in a low wide-mouth jar.

MOISTURIZER FOR AROUND THE MOUTH

Don't ignore the skin around your lips. Due to a variety of factors, small lines can appear around the lip area. An application of this moisturizer can help to soften lines and give a more youthful appearance.

> 1 tsp. jojoba oil
> ¼ tsp. evening primrose oil
> 800 IU Vitamin E
> 1 drop carrot seed essential oil
> 1 drop frankincense essential oil

Mix all of the ingredients together well. Store in a small bottle with a tightly fitting cap. Massage a drop or two to the skin around your lips once a day.

Mouth and Tooth Care

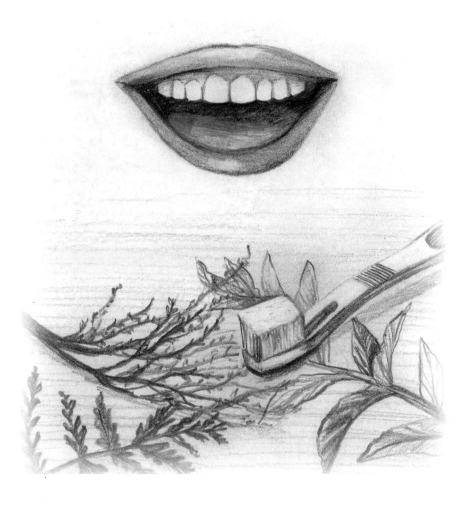

There are several natural alternatives to commercial toothpaste preparations. My recipes include some classic tooth cleaning ingredients such as baking soda and/or table salt. Mouth freshening preparations are as close as your herb bed or spice cabinet.

OTHER TIPS FOR GOOD
MOUTH CARE

§ *Eating foods with a high refined sugar content can increase the likelihood of bad breath. For fresher breath, decrease your intake of these foods.*

§ *Using a soft bristle toothbrush decreases the chance of harming gums and other soft tissues in the mouth.*

§ *Try this simple mechanical way to freshen your mouth—brush your tongue when your brush your teeth—it really helps to decrease mouth odor.*

§ *Coffee, tea, and tobacco products can stain your teeth. For whiter teeth, avoid the use of these products.*

BAKING SODA-THYME TOOTH CLEANER

This preparation has a medicinal taste that is not unpleasant. Your mouth will feel very fresh after you use this product.

1 tsp. baking soda
1 drop thyme essential oil

Mix the essential oil into the baking soda. Dampen a toothbrush with water, dip into the tooth cleaner, and brush your teeth as usual.

BAKING SODA-PEPPERMINT TOOTH CLEANER

Fresh and pleasant tasting!

> ¼ tsp. table salt
> ¼ tsp. baking soda
> 1 drop peppermint essential oil

Mix all of the ingredients together. Dampen a toothbrush with water, dip into the tooth cleaner, and brush your teeth as usual.

BAKING SODA-MYRRH TOOTH CLEANER

Myrrh essential oil is a tried and true ingredient for mouth and gum care. This preparation gives your mouth an invigorating feel.

> 1 tsp. table salt
> t tsp. baking soda
> 2 drops myrrh essential oil

Mix all of the ingredients together. Dampen a toothbrush with water, dip into the mixture, and brush your teeth as usual.

BAKING SODA-CLOVE TOOTH CLEANER

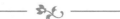

This cleaner has a spicy-clean feel and fragrance.

> ½ tsp. baking soda
> ½ tsp. table salt
> 1 drop clove essential oil

Mix all of the ingredients together. Dampen a toothbrush with water, dip into the mixture, and brush your teeth as usual.

FULLER'S EARTH ORAL
ODOR-EATER

Clay is absorbent and helps to reduce mouth odor.

¼ tsp. baking soda
⅛ tsp. fuller's earth
1 drop myrrh essential oil

Mix all of the ingredients together. Dampen a toothbrush with water, dip into the mixture, and brush your teeth as usual.

KAOLIN TOOTH WHITENER

This recipe has a naturally sweet taste from the vegetable glycerine and the gently abrasive action of the kaolin helps to whiten teeth.

1 tsp. kaolin
1 tsp. vegetable glycerine

Mix the two ingredients together. Place on a dampened toothbrush and brush your teeth as usual.

CINNAMON-CLOVE MOUTHWASH

The exotic spices leave your mouth feeling clean and fresh.

- ¾ cup distilled water
- 1 Tbsp. pure grain alcohol or good quality vodka
- 1 drop clove essential oil
- 1 drop myrrh essential oil
- 1 drop cinnamon essential oil

Add the essential oils to the alcohol and mix well. Add the distilled water. This will turn into a cloudy looking fluid. Use a tablespoon of the mixture at a time as a mouthwash. Store in a bottle with a tight lid. This will last for 5-6 weeks.

PEPPERMINT-MYRRH MOUTHWASH

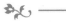

Peppermint is a classic addition to mouthwash and myrrh essential oil lends a healing quality to this recipe.

- ½ cup distilled water
- 1 Tbsp. pure grain alcohol or good quality vodka
- 1 drop peppermint essential oil
- 1 drop myrrh essential oil

Add the essential oils to the alcohol and mix well. Add the distilled water. This will turn into a cloudy looking fluid. Use a tablespoon at a time as a mouthwash. Store in a bottle with a tight lid. This solution will keep for 5-6 weeks.

WARM N' SPICY MOUTHWASH

This mouthwash has a very strong spicy flavor.

   1 cup distilled water
   2 Tbsp. pure grain alcohol or good quality vodka
   ½ tsp. ground cloves
   ½ tsp. ground cinnamon
   ½ tsp. fennel seeds

Mix the spices into the alcohol. Cover and let the mixture sit for three days. Strain the spices from the alcohol by pouring through a paper coffee filter placed in a strainer. Add the distilled water to the strained mixture. It will turn cloudy. Use a tablespoon at a time as a mouthwash. Store in a bottle with a tight lid. This solution will keep for 5-6 weeks.

PARSLEY MOUTH FRESHENER

Chew and swallow a sprig of fresh parsley. It will freshen your breath due to the high chlorophyll content in the parsley. (Now you know why restaurants put parsley on your plate. It's not just for garnish!)

FENNEL MOUTH FRESHENER

Chew ½ tsp. fennel seeds, then swallow them or spit them out, whichever you prefer. Fennel seeds have a strong licorice flavor that is freshening to your breath.

DILL MOUTH FRESHENER

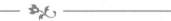

Chew ½ tsp. dill seeds, then swallow them or spit them out, whichever you prefer. Dill seeds have a spicy flavor that freshens your breath.

PEPPERMINT MOUTH FRESHENER

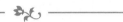

Chew one or two peppermint leaves, then swallow them or spit them out, whichever you prefer. As most of us know, peppermint is a great breath freshener.

Hand Cleansers

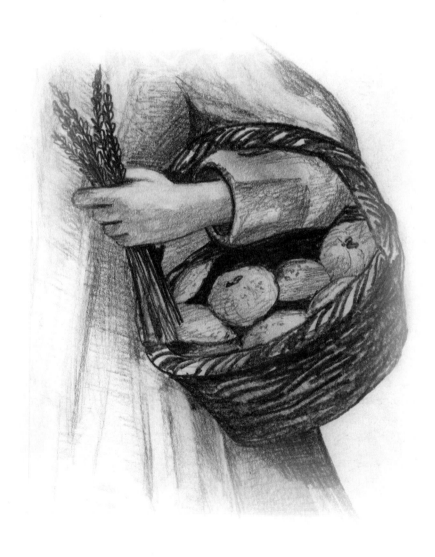

HEAVY DUTY CLEANER

This easy method of cleaning hands has been used around our house for removing everything from heavy grease and grime to the sticky resin from evergreen trees that clings to your skin. Not only does it clean, but it moisturizes and softens your hands as well.

Rub 1-2 teaspoons of wheat germ oil into your hands, then wipe off the excess oil and dirt with a damp cloth or paper towel.

CITRUS CLEANER

This treatment not only cleans your hands but helps to remove any odors. What could be simpler?

Cut one fresh lemon in half. Rub the cut side of the lemon onto your hands, squeezing the lemon a bit to extract some of the juice. Rub the juice into your hands, then rinse with water. Wipe hands dry with a soft cloth or paper towel.

PICNIC CLEANSER

This recipe provides instant cleanup for sticky hands without making an extra trip into the house during picnics or cookouts. This product could also be made up to take with you while traveling. It's an easy way to wash hands and faces when you aren't near a source of water.

> **2 cups water**
> **1 tsp. pure grain alcohol or good quality vodka**
> **2-3 drops of lemon, lime, orange, OR tangerine essential oil, your choice**
> **Sturdy paper towels**

Add your choice of essential oil to the alcohol. Add the essential oil/alcohol mixture to the water and stir. Moisten sturdy paper towels in the mixture and place in a plastic bag for use when needed. To use, wipe a moistened paper towel on dirty hands or faces and let them air dry. Any of the mixture that is leftover can be stored in a bottle. Label the bottle with its contents.

Variation: Store the cleanser in a plastic squeeze bottle labeled with its contents. Squeeze the cleanser onto paper towels immediately before using.

WATERLESS HAND CLEANER

The lemon essential oil in this recipe gives this product a clean fresh smell and the castor oil helps to keep hands soft.

> 2 Tbsp. castor oil
> 1 Tbsp. fuller's earth
> ¼ tsp. liquid dish detergent
> ¼ tsp. tincture of benzoin
> 3 drops lemon essential oil

Mix all of the ingredients together. Place them in a low wide mouth jar. To use, rub about 1 teaspoon of the mixture onto dirty hands, then wipe off with a damp soft cloth or paper towel.

CREAMY SOAP IN A JAR

Keep a jar of this at the kitchen sink for quick hand cleaning. This recipe can be used as a body soap in the bath or shower as well.

> 1 cup distilled water
> ½ cup grated pure or Castile soap
> 1 Tbsp. witch hazel extract
> 1 Tbsp. sweet almond oil
> 3 drops lavender essential oil
> pinch borax

Heat the distilled water in a saucepan. Add the borax to the water and stir until the borax is dissolved. Add the grated soap to the water and bring to a boil, stirring gently until the soap has dissolved. Remove the mixture from the heat. Whisk in the witch hazel extract and the sweet almond oil. Allow the mixture to cool slightly, then mix in the lavender essential oil. For a fluffier mixture, whisk it some more. Store in a low wide-mouthed jar. To use, spoon out about 1 teaspoonful of the soap on your hands, add water, and wash as usual.

HANDWASHING SOAP

This soap is appropriate for use in the kitchen and bath.

½ cup distilled water
¼ cup grated pure soap
¼ cup witch hazel extract
¾ tsp. arrowroot powder
15 drops grapefruit seed extract
5 drops lemon essential oil

Bring the distilled water to a boil in a saucepan. Add the grated soap, lower the heat, and simmer until the soap is dissolved, stirring occasionally. Add the arrowroot powder and whisk until it is mixed into the soap and water. Continue to heat on low for about 15 minutes and whisk frequently. Remove the mixture from the heat source. Add the witch hazel extract and grapefruit seed extract and stir. Allow the mixture to cool slightly, then add the essential oil. Stir the mixture occasionally while it is cooling to prevent it from separating. Store in a low wide-mouth jar. To use, spoon out about 1 teaspoonful of the soap on your hands, add water, and wash as usual.

Hand Creams

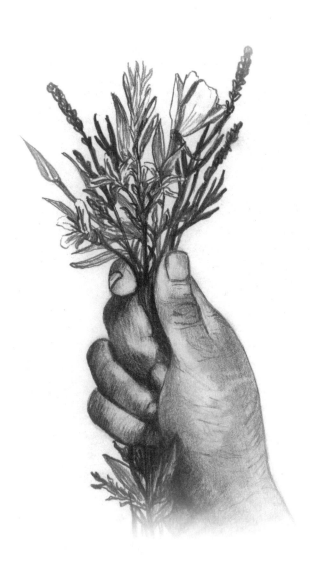

$\mathcal{S}$peaking for myself, I find that my hands take a lot of abuse from work and exposure to the elements. When developing these recipes, I was especially trying to make products that are protective, softening, and healing when needed. It is my opinion that you will find that these products meet all of these needs. Any of the following preparations can be used on the body as well as on the hands.

GENERAL GUIDELINES
FOR MAKING CREAMS

§ *If the consistency of any of the following products does not please you, use these instructions for adjusting the ingredients to achieve the results that you want.*

To thin preparations: *Add more oil in increments of one teaspoon at a time until it reaches the consistency that you desire.*

To thicken preparations: *Add more beeswax in increments of ½ teaspoon at a time until it reaches the consistency that you desire.*

§ *It takes preparations made with shea butter longer to cool and return to a solid/semi-solid consistency.*

§ *In rare instances, some of the oil in certain recipes will separate out of the finished product. Simply stir the preparation before using to mix the ingredients back together.*

§ *Always add the essential oils at the end of the process while the mixture is cooling.*

§ *Any of the finished creams can be placed in storage containers before they completely cool.*

§ CAUTION: *Ingredients melted over boiling water will be very hot. To prevent burns, use hot pads or mitts to remove the heat proof container from the boiling water and avoid skin contact with the melted ingredients until they have cooled.*

CREAMY HONEY

This preparation is a rich golden color with lots of ingredients that will help to maintain your skin's integrity. Thank the hard working honeybee for some of the ingredients in this recipe!

- 1 Tbsp. beeswax (pearls or solid beeswax grated and measured)
- 1 Tbsp. shea butter
- 1 Tbsp. wheat germ oil
- 2 tsp. honey
- ½ tsp. rosehip seed oil
- 800 IU Vitamin E
- 2 drops lemon essential oil
- 2 drops sandalwood essential oil
- 2 drops geranium essential oil

Place the beeswax, shea butter, and wheat germ oil in a heat proof container. Melt the ingredients over boiling water. Remove the mixture from the heat source when the ingredients have melted. Whisk in the honey, rosehip seed oil, and Vitamin E. Occasionally whisk the mixture as it cools. When it is cooling, add the essential oils and mix well. Store in a low wide-mouth jar.

AVOCADO HAND CREAM

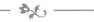

The richness of avocado oil makes your skin feel very soft. This recipe is my husband's favorite. He uses it on a daily basis to keep his hands soft and trouble-free.

1 Tbsp. avocado oil
1 tsp. beeswax (pearls or solid beeswax grated and measured)
1 tsp. jojoba oil
20 drops evening primrose oil
800 IU Vitamin E
5 drops carrot seed essential oil
3 drops patchouli essential oil
2 drops frankincense essential oil
1 drop rosewood essential oil

Place the beeswax and avocado oil in a heat proof container. Melt the ingredients over boiling water. When melted, remove from the heat source. Add the evening primrose oil, jojoba oil, and Vitamin E and mix thoroughly. When the mixture is cooling, mix in the essential oils. Store in a low wide-mouth jar.

SOFTEN YOUR HANDS CREAM

I gave some of this recipe to my 89 year old friend to try. She loved the aroma and creamy consistency of this preparation.

1 Tbsp. shea butter
1 tsp. coconut oil
½ tsp. wheat germ oil
½ tsp. vegetable glycerine
15 drops grapefruit seed extract
400 IU Vitamin E
6 drops lavender essential oil
6 drops geranium essential oil

Mix the vegetable glycerine and grapefruit seed extract in a separate container and set aside. Place the shea butter, coconut oil, and wheat germ oil in a heat proof container and melt over boiling water. When the mixture has melted, remove it from the heat source. Add the Vitamin E and glycerine/grapefruit seed extract mixture and combine with the melted ingredients using a whisk. While the preparation is cooling add the essential oils and mix them in thoroughly. Store in a low wide-mouth jar.

MY OWN HAND CREAM

"What makes this so smooth?" asked my mother after she tried it. The secret is the shea butter, which gives any preparation a lovely creamy consistency. This cream can be used on the skin on all parts of your body with satisfactory results.

2 Tbsp. shea butter
1 Tbsp. apricot kernel oil
1 tsp. avocado oil
½ tsp. rosehip seed oil
½ tsp. rosewater or rose hydrosol
800 IU Vitamin E
6 drops lavender essential oil

Place the shea butter, apricot kernel oil, and avocado oil in a heat proof container and melt over boiling water. When the mixture has melted, remove it from the heat source. Add the rosehip seed oil and Vitamin E and whisk. While the mixture is cooling, add the rosewater and the essential oil. Store in a low wide-mouth jar.

HEALING HAND CREAM

This heavy duty cream is very thick. With the many soothing ingredients, it is useful for chapped irritated hands.

2 Tbsp. castor oil
1 Tbsp. wheat germ oil
2 tsp. beeswax (pearls or solid beeswax grated and measured)
15 drops grapefruit seed extract
10 drops jojoba oil
½ tsp. liquid lecithin
800 IU Vitamin E
4 drops myrrh essential oil
4 drops tea tree essential oil
3 drops German chamomile essential oil

Place the beeswax, castor oil, and wheat germ oil in a heat proof container and melt over boiling water. Remove the mixture from the heat source when it is melted. Add the jojoba oil and Vitamin E and whisk together. Add the liquid lecithin and grapefruit seed extract. Stir all of the ingredients together with a whisk. While the mixture is cooling, add the essential oils and mix well. Store in a low wide-mouth jar.

RICHLY SCENTED HAND CREAM

Add this cream to any pampering ritual that you may have. Its rich scent is truly luxurious. One of my friends has dry, very sensitive skin and used it on her face without any problems.

2 Tbsp. shea butter
1 Tbsp. avocado oil
1 Tbsp. rosewater or rose hydrosol
1 tsp. rosehip seed oil
1 tsp. liquid lecithin
800 IU Vitamin E
5 drops ylang ylang essential oil
4 drops lemon essential oil
2 drops patchouli essential oil

Place the shea butter and avocado oil in a heat proof container and melt over boiling water. After it has melted, remove it from the heat source. Add the rosehip seed oil, Vitamin E, and liquid lecithin. Whisk all of the ingredients thoroughly. Add the rosewater and mix thoroughly. As the preparation is cooling, add the essential oils and mix. Store in a low wide-mouth jar.

"NOT JUST FOR BABY" CREAM

This cream is safe to use on a baby's tender skin and can be used as a diaper cream. Don't forget to use it on grownup skin, too!

> 3½ Tbsp. castor oil
> 2 Tbsp. beeswax (pearls or solid beeswax grated and measured)
> 1 Tbsp. sweet almond oil
> 10 drops jojoba oil
> 800 IU Vitamin E
> 1 drop German chamomile essential oil
> 1 drop lavender essential oil

Place the beeswax, castor oil, and sweet almond oil in a heat proof container and heat over boiling water. When the beeswax has melted into the oils, remove them from the heat source. Add the jojoba oil and Vitamin E and mix well with a whisk. While the mixture is cooling, add the essential oils and mix thoroughly. Store in a low wide-mouth jar.

COLD CREAM

This cream can be used to remove makeup as well as for a general facial and body moisturizer. One of my friends applies this cream to her face and lets the heat from her shower soak the moisturizing properties into her skin during the process. She then removes it at the end of her shower and tells me, "It keep my winter skin soft and moist."

3 Tbsp. olive oil
1 Tbsp. aloe vera gel
1 Tbsp. shea butter
1 Tbsp. rosewater or rose hydrosol
2 tsp. beeswax (pearls or solid beeswax grated and measured)
¼ tsp. liquid lecithin
800 IU Vitamin E
3 drops German chamomile essential oil

In a separate container, mix the aloe vera gel and rosewater and set aside. Place the olive oil, shea butter, and beeswax together in a heat proof container over boiling water. Remove from the heat source after the mixture has melted. Add the Vitamin E and liquid lecithin and mix well. Combine this mixture with the aloe vera gel and rosewater mixture. Stir with a whisk to combine thoroughly. While the mixture is cooling, add the essential oil. Store in a low wide-mouth jar.

LIGHT CREAM

The addition of calendula infused oil add a therapeutic touch to this recipe. One of my friends had surgery and came home with "sheet burns" on her elbows. She applied this cream to her elbows to aid in the healing process.

1 Tbsp. coconut oil
1 Tbsp. rosewater or rose hydrosol
2 tsp. beeswax (pearls or solid beeswax grated and measured)
2 tsp. calendula infused oil (See instructions for making this in the
    Body and Bath Oil section of this book.)
2 tsp. vegetable glycerine
¼ tsp. liquid lecithin
800 IU Vitamin E
10 drops carrot seed essential oil
5 drops rosewood essential oil
2 drops frankincense essential oil

In a separate container combine the vegetable glycerine and rosewater and set aside. Place the beeswax, coconut oil, and calendula oil together in a heat proof container over boiling water. Remove the mixture from the heat source when it has melted. Add the liquid lecithin and Vitamin E and mix well. While whisking the mixture, add the combined rosewater and vegetable glycerine. While the mixture is cooling, add the essential oils and mix thoroughly. Store in a low wide-mouth jar.

APRICOT HAND CREAM

1½ Tbsp. vegetable glycerine
1½ Tbsp. coconut oil
1 Tbsp. apricot kernel oil
2 tsp. beeswax (pearls or solid beeswax grated and measured)
800 IU Vitamin E
3 drops bergamot essential oil

Place the beeswax, apricot kernel oil, and coconut oil in a heat proof container and melt over boiling water. Remove from the heat source when the mixture is melted. Add the vitamin E and mix well using a whisk. Add the vegetable glycerine slowly, whisking continually as it is added. While the mixture is cooling, add the essential oil and mix to blend. Store in a low wide-mouth jar.

HERBAL-LEMON MOISTURIZER

1 Tbsp. sweet almond oil
1 Tbsp. coconut oil
1 Tbsp rosewater or rose hydrosol
1 Tbsp. vegetable glycerine
1 Tbsp. aloe vera gel
2 tsp. beeswax (pearls or solid beeswax grated and measured)
1 tsp. avocado oil
1 tsp. apricot kernel oil
¼ tsp. liquid lecithin
800 IU Vitamin E
6 drops lemon essential oil

In a separate container, mix the vegetable glycerine, rosewater, and aloe vera gel and set aside. Place the beeswax, sweet almond oil, coconut oil, avocado oil, and apricot kernel oil in a heat proof container and melt over boiling water. After the mixture is melted, remove from the heat source. Add the liquid lecithin and Vitamin E to the mixture, stirring well with a whisk. Slowly add the glycerine/rosewater/aloe vera gel mixture to the rest of the ingredients, stirring well with a whisk while adding. While the mixture is cooling, add the essential oil. Store in a low wide-mouth container.

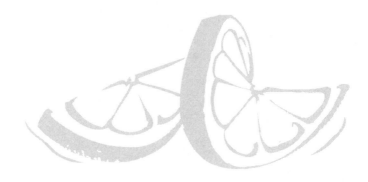

"BUTTERY" RICH BODY BALM

The richness of shea butter and cocoa butter combine in this recipe to make a wonderful body cream.

> 1 Tbsp. shea butter
> 2 tsp. cocoa butter
> 2 tsp. apricot kernel oil
> 1 tsp. aloe vera gel
> 800 IU Vitamin E
> ¼ tsp. liquid lecithin
> 5 drops grapefruit seed extract
> 3 drops lemon essential oil
> 3 drops geranium essential oil

In a separate container, mix the aloe vera gel and grapefruit seed extract and set aside. Place the shea butter, cocoa butter, and apricot kernel oil in a heat proof container and melt over boiling water. Remove from the heat source when the ingredients are melted. Add the Vitamin E and the liquid lecithin, mixing well. Whisk in the aloe vera gel and grapefruit seed extract. While the mixture is cooling, add the essential oils. Store in a low wide-mouth jar.

MY FAVORITE INGREDIENTS FORMULA

It stands to reason that you will have some ingredients that stand out as your favorites when you make recipes. This recipe is the combination of some of the ones that I like best.

2 Tbsp. shea butter
1 Tbsp. avocado oil
1 tsp. rosewater or rose hydrosol
½ tsp. beeswax (pearls or solid beeswax grated and measured)
¼ tsp. liquid lecithin
10 drops grapefruit seed extract
800 IU Vitamin E
5 drops carrot seed essential oil
4 drops lavender essential oil
3 drops German chamomile essential oil
2 drops lemon essential oil

In a separate container, mix the rosewater and grapefruit seed extract and set aside. Place the shea butter, avocado oil, and beeswax in a heat proof container and melt over boiling water. Remove the mixture from the heat source when it has melted. Add the Vitamin E and liquid lecithin and whisk together. Add the rosewater/grapefruit seed extract mixture to the rest of the ingredients and mix thoroughly using a whisk. While the mixture is cooling, add the essential oils and mix well. Store in a low wide-mouth jar.

Natural Beauty Basics

DAILY HAND CARE CREAM

This is thick, rich, and absorbs easily into the skin.

1 Tbsp. shea butter
2 tsp. beeswax (pearls or solid beeswax grated and measured)
2 tsp. avocado oil
2 tsp. vegetable glycerine
1 tsp. cocoa butter
¼ tsp. liquid lecithin
800 IU Vitamin E
2 drops German chamomile essential oil
2 drops lavender essential oil
1 drop rosemary essential oil

Place the beeswax, shea butter, cocoa butter, and avocado oil in a heat proof container and melt over boiling water. Remove from the heat source when the ingredients have melted. Add the Vitamin E and liquid lecithin to the mixture. Slowly add the vegetable glycerine, mixing with a whisk continually. While the mixture is cooling, add the essential oils and mix well. Store in a low wide-mouth jar.

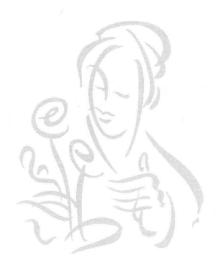

CALENDULA CREAM

Skin that is troubled and irritated can benefit from the healing properties of ca-lendula.

> 1 Tbsp. calendula infused oil (See instructions for making in the
>   Body and Bath Oil section of this book.)
> 1 Tbsp. avocado oil
> 1 Tbsp. coconut oil
> 1 tsp. beeswax (pearls or solid beeswax grated and measured)
> 20 drops jojoba oil
> 800 IU Vitamin E
> 5 drops carrot seed essential oil
> 5 drops lemon essential oil
> 3 drops rosemary essential oil

Place the beeswax, calendula infused oil, avocado oil, and coconut oil in a heat proof container and melt over boiling water. Remove from the heat source when the ingredients have melted. Add the jojoba oil and Vitamin E to the mixture, using a whisk to mix well. While the mixture is cooling add the essential oils and mix thoroughly. Store in a low wide-mouth jar.

PROTECTIVE LOTION

This thick liquid preparation is good to put on your hands before you expose them to cold wet conditions. The lanolin serves as a protective barrier and the cocoa butter is moisturizing.

> 2 tsp. castor oil
> 1½ tsp. cocoa butter
> 1 tsp. lanolin
> 800 IU Vitamin E
> 5 drops lavender essential oil
> 3 drops tea tree essential oil

Place the castor oil, cocoa butter, and lanolin in a heat proof container and melt over boiling water. Remove from the heat source when all of the ingredients have melted. Whisk the Vitamin E into the mixture. While the mixture is cooling, add the essential oils and mix well. Store in a bottle or jar.

HERBAL CREAM

2 tsp. calendula infused oil
1 tsp. German chamomile infused oil
(See instructions for making both infused oils in the Body and Bath
   Oil section of this book.)
2 tsp. beeswax (pearls or solid beeswax grated and measured)
1 tsp. castor oil
1 tsp. aloe vera gel
¼ tsp. liquid lecithin
800 IU Vitamin E
5 drops carrot seed essential oil
4 drops orange essential oil
2 drops rosemary essential oil
2 drops rosewood essential oil

Place the infused oils, beeswax, and castor oil in a heat proof container and melt over boiling water. Remove from the heat source when all of the ingredients have melted. Add the Vitamin E and liquid lecithin and mix well. Add the aloe vera gel and mix well. While the mixture is cooling, add the essential oils and mix thoroughly. Store in a low wide-mouth jar.

SHEA BUTTER CREAM

This is one of the creams that I like to take with me when traveling.

1 Tbsp. shea butter
1 tsp. avocado oil
½ tsp. beeswax (pearls or solid beeswax grated and measured)
800 IU Vitamin E
6 drops carrot seed essential oil
4 drops geranium essential oil
1 drop rosemary essential oil

Place the shea butter, beeswax, and avocado oil in a heat proof container and melt over boiling water. After it has melted, remove the mixture from the heat source and add the Vitamin E, mixing well. While the mixture is cooling, add the essential oils and mix thoroughly. Store in a low wide-mouth jar.

Sleep Pillows

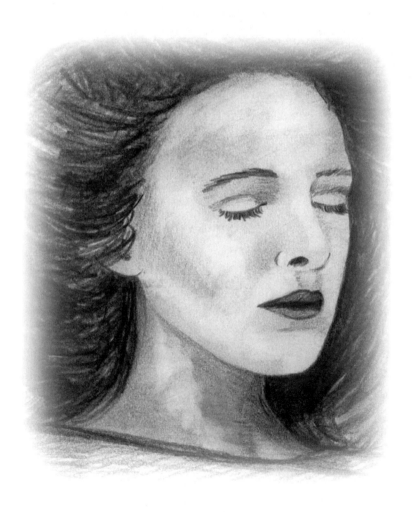

he aroma of these little pillows can help to lull you to sleep on one of those nights when you are tossing and turning. These are not full-sized pillows. Instead, these small cloth covered packages containing dried herbs and other ingredients are meant to be tucked between your bed pillow and its pillowcase. Rest your head on it to help release the aromas. For gift giving or as a treat to yourself, "fancy up" these gems with special fabric, laces, and ribbons.

All of these recipes call for cellulose chips as a fixative for the essential oils. In recipes in other sources orris root is frequently called for as a fixative agent. Many people, myself included, have severe headaches when exposed to it. As a consequence of this reaction, I avoid using it whenever possible.

SLEEP PILLOW

Hops is typically thought of as an ingredient for brewing beer. Since it is reported to contain a substance that helps to induce sleep, it is appropriately used here as the primary ingredient.

> ½ **cup dried hops**
> ¼ **cup dried lemon verbena leaves**
> ¼ **cup dried lavender buds**
> **2 Tbsp. cellulose chips**
> **4 drops lemon essential oil**
> **4 drops lavender essential oil**
> **Two fabric pillows 6 inches square, each with one end open**

In a glass bowl or measuring cup, mix the essential oils into the cellulose chips. Cover and set aside for four hours or more. The longer you let these two ingredients blend, the longer lasting the aroma from the essential oils will be. Mix in the dried herbs. Place half of the mixture into each fabric pillow and sew or fasten the open end closed.

LAVENDER SLEEP PILLOW

The fragrances of lavender and bergamot in this recipe are very pleasant. Sweet dreams!

1 cup dried hops
1 cup dried lavender buds
¼ cup dried thyme leaves
3 Tbsp. cellulose chips
10 drops lavender essential oil
10 drops bergamot essential oil
Two fabric pillows 6 inches square, each with one end open

In a glass bowl or measuring cup, mix the essential oils into the cellulose chips. Cover and set aside overnight. The next day mix in the dried herbs. Place half of the mixture into each fabric pillow and sew or fasten the open end closed.

STORING LEFTOVERS

If you have more of the dried mixture than will fit into your fabric pillows, store in a glass jar away from direct heat and light. Label the jar with its contents. You could also place the dried mixture in an open container and put it in your bedroom, using it much as you would a potpourri mixture.

SWEET DREAMS SLEEP PILLOW

The essential oils and German chamomile blossoms lend a sweet floral scent to this mixture.

1 cup dried hops
½ cup dried German chamomile blossoms
2 Tbsp. cellulose chips
2 drops geranium essential oil
2 drops ylang ylang essential oil
Two fabric pillows 6 inches square, each with one end open

In a glass bowl or measuring cup, mix the essential oils into the cellulose chips. Cover and set aside overnight. Mix the dried herbs into the bowl, then use half of the mixture in each fabric pillow. Sew or fasten the open end closed.

AROMATIC SLEEP PILLOW

The aroma of the catnip and the rosemary essential oil will aid in opening up your sinuses if you are suffering from a cold.

¼ cup dried hops
¼ cup dried catnip leaves
¼ cup dried lemon balm leaves
¼ cup cellulose chips
2 Tbsp. dried lavender buds
6 drops rosemary essential oil
3 drops lavender essential oil
Two fabric pillows 6 inches square, each with one end open

In a glass bowl or measuring cup, mix the essential oils into the cellulose chips. Cover and set aside overnight. Mix in the dried herbs and use half of the mixture in each fabric pillow. Sew or fasten the open end closed.

Variation: Substitute dried rosemary leaves for the lemon balm leaves.

RELAXING ESSENTIAL OILS

In addition to the essential oils used in this section's recipes, each of the following essential oils have the reputation for having a relaxing aroma and are also good choices for additions to a sleep pillow recipe.

clary sage	*basil*	*myrrh*
German chamomile	*neroli*	*orange*
patchouli	*sandalwood*	*frankincense*
rose	*tangerine*	*cedarwood*

RELAX AND REST PILLOW

The lavender and lemon aroma in this recipe leaves most people pleasantly relaxed. See what you think.

> **1 cup dried lemon balm leaves**
> **¼ cup dried lavender buds**
> **3 Tbsp. cellulose chips**
> **6 drops lemon essential oil**
> **2 drops lavender essential oil**
> **one fabric pillow 6 inches square with one end open**

In a glass bowl or measuring cup, mix the essential oils into the cellulose chips. Cover and set aside overnight. Mix in the dried herbs and place the mixture into the fabric pillow. Sew or fasten the open end closed.

Body Powder

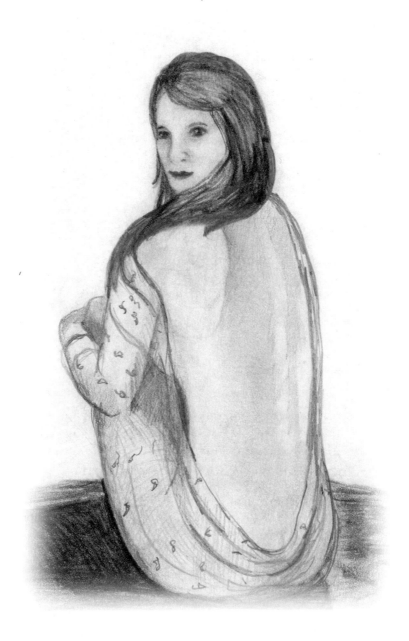

While experimenting, I found that many body powder recipes from other sources produce a clumpy product that won't easily shake from a container. The secret to a smooth powder that shakes easily from a container is the addition of clay. The texture is not only improved, but the absorbency is enhanced.

Many commercial powders contain talc, potentially irritating to the lungs. Although the small particles of any of the ingredients in these recipes can also be irritating to the lungs, they are less so than talc. To decrease the chance of lung irritation, avoid inhaling the powder when it is applied and don't generate a cloud of powder when applying it.

Using shaker containers for powder applications is the best way to avoid the bacterial contamination that can occur when using powder puffs. Shake the powder onto your hand and smooth it on the body where desired, or shake the powder directly onto your body.

FLORAL BODY POWDER

This powder has a floral scent. It can keep you feeling fresh all day!

- 1 Tbsp. arrowroot powder
- 1 Tbsp. kaolin
- 1 Tbsp. baking soda
- 3 drops geranium essential oil
- 2 drops jasmine essential oil

In a glass bowl or measuring cup, mix all of the dry ingredients together. Add the essential oils and mix well. Cover the container and set aside for several hours to give the essential oils time to absorb into the dry ingredients. Put the finished product into a shaker container.

Variation: Substitute five drops of any essential oil or a combination of two essential oils for a desired fragrance. Do not exceed five drops total of essential oil for the above recipe.

SWEET SMELLING POWDER

1 cup arrowroot powder
¼ cup baking soda
¼ cup clay (fuller's earth, kaolin, or green clay, your choice)
7 drops lavender essential oil
7 drops orange essential oil
2 drops lemon essential oil

In a glass bowl or measuring cup, mix all of the dry ingredients together. Add the essential oils and mix well. Cover the container and set aside for several hours to give the essential oils time to absorb into the dry ingredients. Put the finished product in a shaker container.

CHAMOMILE POWDER

This is a soothing recipe with the German chamomile blossoms and essential oil as ingredients.

1 cup arrowroot powder
¼ cup kaolin
¼ cup baking soda
1 Tbsp. ground and sifted German chamomile blossoms
8 drops orange essential oil
4 drops German chamomile essential oil

Mix all of the ingredients together thoroughly in a glass bowl or measuring cup. Cover and set aside overnight. Put the finished product in a shaker container.

Variation: Substitute ground and sifted dried lavender buds and lavender essential oil for the German chamomile blossoms and essential oil. Combine the rest of the ingredients as directed.

BENTONITE POWDER

Bentonite clay is highly absorbent and recommended for use on areas of the skin where moisture can be trapped. Tea tree essential oil's healing properties could qualify this recipe as a "medicated" powder.

¾ **cup bentonite clay**
¼ **cup kaolin**
12 drops tea tree essential oil
5 drops lavender essential oil

Mix all of the ingredients in a glass bowl or measuring cup. Cover and set aside overnight. Put the finished product in a shaker container.

Bath Time

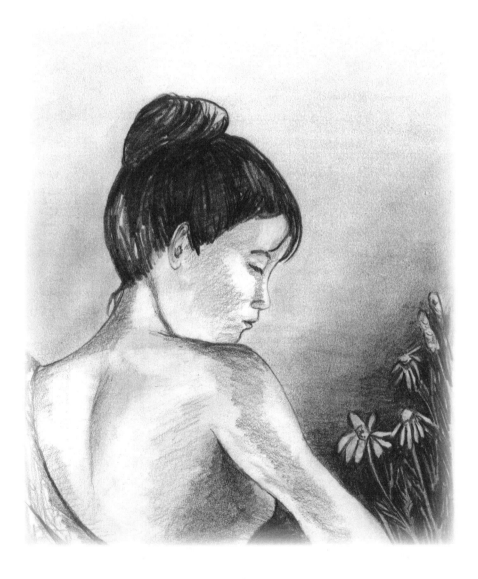

$\mathcal{E}$veryone has seen the pictures of people luxuriating in a bathtub filled to the brim with foamy suds and candles surrounding them. An inviting scene to be sure, but it isn't something that many of us get to do very often. However, 15 minutes of your time set aside once in a while for a relaxing bath isn't out of reach for most of us. A good soak can soothe your nerves and soften the skin. Set this short amount of time aside once in a while for this special activity. You'll be glad that you did.

BATH BAG HERBS

If you can't find the little muslin tea bags for this recipe, use a clean sock that doesn't have a mate. (Who doesn't have one of those in their laundry room?) Either the muslin tea bag or clean sock can be rinsed and dried and used many times.

> 1 Tbsp. dried lavender buds
> 1 Tbsp. dried rosemary
> 1 Tbsp. dried mint, your choice
> 1 Tbsp. dried German chamomile blossoms
> 1 muslin tea bag or clean sock

Mix the dried herbs together and place in the muslin tea bag or clean sock. Close either of these tightly. The muslin tea bag comes with a drawstring, or you can tie the end of the sock closed. Place the bag in a saucepan with 1 quart of water. Bring the water to a boil and simmer for 10 minutes. Remove the saucepan from the heat, and allow the mixture to cool to room temperature. Add the bag of herbs and the infusion to a tub of warm water. Soak in the tub, using the bag of herbs as a washcloth.

Variations: This recipe just begs to be changed according to what dried herbs you have available or what aroma you want. Substitute any dried herb in this recipe, using the same amounts as noted. Some suggested combinations are:

- HEALING MIX: calendula, thyme, lemon balm, lemon verbena

- SKIN SOFTENING MIX: fennel seeds, parsley, rosemary, German chamomile

- DEODORIZING MIX: basil, lavender, rosemary, sage

- FLORAL MIX: lavender, rose petals, German chamomile, lemon balm

- SKIN TONING MIX: lady's mantle, rosemary, yarrow, lemon verbena

- RELAXING MIX: lemon balm, lavender, catnip, German chamomile

- SLEEPY TIME MIX: hops, lavender, catnip, lemon verbena

OR: Substitute any single dried herb that you desire. Use 4 tablespoons (¼ cup) of any single dried herb.

OR: Combine the benefits of any two herbs in the recipe. Use 2 tablespoons of each one.

FOR THOSE WHO CAN'T TAKE BATHS

Taking a bath may not be an option for you if you are unable to get in and out of a bathtub due to physical limitations, or you are prone to urinary tract infections. To benefit from the effects of the ingredients in any of these recipes that call for using a bath bag, simply use the bag filled with any bath mixture in the shower as a washcloth. Wet the bag in the running water frequently as you use it. For the Bath Bag Herb recipe, reserve the infusion to use as an after shower body splash.

SOOTHING BATH

Oatmeal is very soothing to all skin types. It is especially good in baths or showers if you suffer from dry, irritated, and/or itchy skin.

2 Tbsp. ground oatmeal
5 drops essential oil, your choice
muslin tea bag or clean sock

Mix the essential oil into the oatmeal. Place in a muslin tea bag or clean sock, and fasten either shut. Fill your bathtub with warm water, keeping the bag under the faucet while the tub is filling. Use the bag as a washcloth.

SUMMER BATH

This mixture is cooling to the skin, making it a good choice for summer use. Of course, it can also be used at other times of the year if you wish!

> 1 Tbsp. dried mint, your choice
> 1 Tbsp. dried lemon peel broken into small pieces
> 2 Tbsp. dried milk powder
> muslin tea bag or clean sock

Place all of the ingredients in the muslin tea bag or clean sock, and fasten either shut. Fill your bathtub with warm water, keeping the bag under the faucet while the tub is filling. Use the bag as a washcloth.

WAKE-UP BATH

The aroma of grapefruit, lavender, and peppermint combine to give you a very awakening feeling. Great when used after a busy day to help revive your senses for evening activities.

> 2 Tbsp. ground oatmeal
> 1 Tbsp. dried lavender buds
> 5 drops grapefruit essential oil
> 2 drops peppermint essential oil
> muslin tea bag or clean sock

Add the essential oils to the oatmeal. Mix the lavender into the oatmeal mixture. Place the mixture into a muslin tea bag or clean sock, and fasten either shut. Fill your bathtub with warm water, keeping the bag under the faucet while the tub is filling. Use the bag as a washcloth.

Variations: One of these uplifting essential oils can be substituted in equal amounts for the grapefruit and peppermint essential oils.

basil   eucalyptus   neroli

geranium   pine   tangerine

INVIGORATING BATH SALTS

The aroma of this recipe seems strong, but once it is diluted in your bath you will find it quite pleasant. Sea salt also has the reputation for drawing impurities from your body.

> 1 cup sea salt, coarse or finely ground (Finely ground will dissolve quicker.)
> 8 drops lime essential oil
> 5 drops eucalyptus essential oil
> 5 drops lavender essential oil
> 4 drops peppermint essential oil
> 2 drops pine essential oil

Place the sea salt in a glass bowl or measuring cup. Add the essential oils and stir into the salt thoroughly. Cover and let the mixture sit for 2 hours, then stir again. Cover and after another 2 hours stir again. Store the bath salts in a glass container with a tight fitting lid.

To use the bath salts, add ½ cup to warm running bath water. Bathe as usual. An alternative: For use in the shower, place 2 tablespoons to ½ cup of the bath salts in a muslin tea bag or clean sock, fastening it tightly. Place the bag in the running shower water, and use it as a washcloth. Wet the bag frequently while you are using it.

Variations: Any mixture of essential oils can be substituted for the essential oils in the recipe. Do not exceed the ratio of 24 drops of essential oil to 1 cup of sea salt.

MILK BATH

Milk baths have been used for centuries by many of history's legendary beauties.

1 cup dried milk powder
10 drops essential oil, your choice

Stir the essential oil into the milk powder. Add the mixture to warm running bath water and bathe as usual. For use in the shower, place ½ cup of the mixture into a muslin tea bag or clean sock, fastening either tightly. Place the bag in the running shower water, and use it as a washcloth. Wet the bag frequently while you are using it. Store any of the leftover mixture in a glass jar with a tight-fitting lid.

WATER SOFTENING BATH

Many parts of the country have hard water full of minerals that can frequently dry out the skin. This recipe will help to soften the water, giving you a gentler bath experience.

½ cup borax
10 drops essential oil, your choice

Mix the essential oil into the borax. For the bath, add 2 tablespoons of the mixture to warm running water, then bathe as usual. Store the remaining mixture in a glass jar with a tight-fitting lid.

BEDTIME BATH

Need to wind down before bedtime? Use this mixture for a relaxing end to your day.

¼ cup finely ground sea salt
6 drops lavender essential oil
2 drops clary sage essential oil
1 drop German chamomile essential oil

Mix the essential oils into the sea salt thoroughly. Pour the mixture into warm running bath water directly under the faucet. Soak for 15 minutes.

Variations: Substitute any of the following relaxing essential oils in equal amounts for the lavender, clary sage, and German chamomile essential oils.

cedarwood	frankincense	myrrh
bergamot	orange	ylang ylang

BATH GIFTS

Making a bath product is an easy and great idea for gift-giving. Follow any of the recipe instructions in this chapter, and place the finished product in an attractive glass jar or other container. Using a ribbon or piece of raffia, tie instructions for the product onto the container with a scoop. Package the gift with a decorative sponge, muslin tea bag, luffa sponge, or pretty washcloth.

BODY REFRESHER SPRAY

Finish off your bath or shower with this recipe. It smells good and makes your skin feel so refreshed. This recipe could also be used as a cologne if you wish.

2 cups distilled water
¼ cup pure grain alcohol or good quality vodka
10 drops essential oils—See the following list for ideas, or make up
    your own combination.

Place the pure grain alcohol or vodka in a glass measuring cup. Add the essential oils. Cover the cup and set it aside for 1 hour. After the hour has passed, add the distilled water and mix well. Put the refresher in spray bottles or decorative narrow necked bottles. (This recipe will fill several 4 ounce containers.) To use, spray or splash on your body where desired, avoiding contact with your eyes.

Possible essential oil combinations for Body Refresher Spray:

- ORANGE BLOSSOM: 8 drops neroli essential oil, 1 drop tangerine essential oil, 1 drop patchouli essential oil

- LAVENDER-LEMON: 8 drops lavender essential oil, 2 drops lemon essential oil

- ROSE-LEMON: 8 drops rose essential oil, 2 drops lemon essential oil

- ROSEMARY-LEMON: 6 drops rosemary essential oil, 4 drops lemon essential oil

SALT BODY SCRUB

The salt not only helps to draw impurities from your body but the coarse texture helps to scrub away dead skin cells, leaving your skin fresh and glowing.

1 cup coarsely ground sea salt
¼ cup olive oil

Stir the olive oil into the sea salt. Standing in the tub or shower, massage 1-2 tablespoons of the scrub over your skin at a time until you have used all of the mixture. Rinse your skin with warm, then cool water.

Variations: Substitute an herbal infused oil for the olive oil. Use the recipe for Infused Oil in the Bath and Body Oil section of this book. Some suggestions are:

- ROSEMARY INFUSED OIL: stimulating, invigorating, deodorizing

- GERMAN CHAMOMILE INFUSED OIL: soothing

- LAVENDER INFUSED OIL: deodorizing

- CALENDULA INFUSED OIL: healing

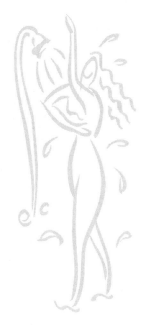

Soaps

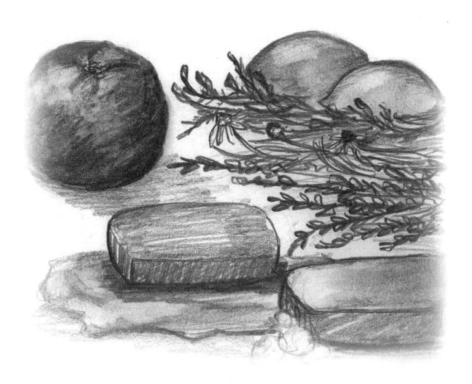

$\mathcal{I}$ have always been intrigued by the idea of making my own soap. However, soap-making recipes intimidate me with the quantity of ingredients involved and the caustic nature of lye that is used in the soap-making process. I have used a method of soap-making that, to my way of thinking, is easier, more economical, and less hazardous. These recipes can be made adding herbs, oils, and essential oils in any combination that strikes my fancy. The type of soap used in these recipes is either pure soap that is made without any additional additives or castile soap that already has some type of vegetable oil in it. Either of these soaps will form a good lather, and work very well in my "cheater" recipes.

HELPFUL HINTS

§ *Soap may be grated ahead of time and stored in recloseable plastic bags. Label the bag with the type of soap that is in each one. This grated soap has an indefinite shelf life and doesn't require any special storage conditions.*

§ *Wet your hands with rosewater or plain water before forming the soap mixture into balls. This prevents the mixture from sticking to your hands and gives the completed balls a smooth shiny finish.*

§ *Pre-grated soap is available for purchase as "rebatchable soap" or "soap curls". See the Resources section in the back of this book for information on companies that sell these products.*

§ *Finished soaps are best wrapped in plastic wrap. They can be stored at room temperature.*

§ *The soap balls have finished drying when there is resistance to moderate pressure on them from your fingers.*

§ *Times vary for the finished soap to dry on waxed paper depending upon the humidity present in your working environment and what size your soap balls are.*

§ *Using ½ cup of each mixture for each soapball is a general guideline. The soapballs can be made whatever size you prefer. Remember that larger soapballs require a longer drying time.*

OATMEAL-LAVENDER SOAP

1 4-ounce bar of pure soap, grated
2 Tbsp. distilled water
2 Tbsp. ground and sifted lavender buds
1 Tbsp. apricot kernel oil
2 tsp. ground oatmeal
3 drops German chamomile essential oil
2 drops lavender essential oil

In a glass bowl or large measuring cup, mix the grated soap, water, and apricot kernel oil. Cover and set aside for one hour, then add the lavender and oatmeal. Stir the ingredients together, then put them into a food processor. Add the essential oils one drop at a time, mixing after each addition. Wet your hands and make the soap into balls, using approximately ½ cup of the mixture for each one. Place the soap balls on waxed paper until dry and firm.

GARDENER'S SOAP

The cornmeal acts as a scrub to clean grimy hands.

1 4-ounce bar of pure soap, grated
2 Tbsp. wheat germ oil
2 tsp. cornmeal
1 tsp. coconut oil
5 drops palmarosa essential oil

Place the soap, wheat germ oil, and coconut oil in a small saucepan. Place the saucepan over low heat and stir frequently until the mixture is "mushy" and blended. (The mixture must be stirred frequently to keep it from scorching.) Remove from the heat and allow the mixture to cool until you can comfortably handle it. Stir in the cornmeal and essential oil and mix well. Wet your hands and form the soap into balls, using approximately ½ cup of the mixture at a time. Place them on waxed paper until they are dry and firm.

LEMON-CALENDULA SOAP

Refreshing aroma and healing qualities combine into one product. It is a useful and enjoyable combination!

> **1 4-ounce bar castile soap, grated**
> **2 Tbsp. rosewater**
> **1 Tbsp. calendula infused oil (See the recipe in the Bath and Body**
>   **Oil section of this book.)**
> **5 drops lemon essential oil**

In a glass bowl or measuring cup, mix the soap, rosewater, and infused oil. Cover and let sit overnight. Place the mixture in a food processor and mix thoroughly. Add the essential oil one drop at a time, mixing well after each addition. Wet your hands and form the soap into balls, using approximately ½ cup of the mixture at a time. Place them on waxed paper until they are dry and firm.

ALOE SOAP

This clean-smelling soap is one of my favorites.

> **1 4-ounce bar castile soap, grated**
> **2 Tbsp. aloe vera gel**
> **1½ Tbsp. rosewater**
> **30 drops evening primrose oil**
> **6 drops tangerine essential oil**
> **4 drops juniper essential oil**

In a glass bowl or measuring cup mix the soap, aloe vera gel, rosewater, and evening primrose oil. Cover and let sit overnight. Place the mixture in a food processor and mix thoroughly. Add the essential oils one drop at a time, mixing well after each addition. Wet your hands and form the soap into balls, using approximately ½ cup of the mixture at a time. Place them on waxed paper until they are dry and firm.

CINNAMON-ROSE-OATMEAL SOAP

The ingredients in this recipe result in a spicy floral fragrance.

1 4-ounce bar castile soap, grated
3 Tbsp. rosewater
2 Tbsp. ground oatmeal
1 Tbsp. sweet almond oil
6 drops cinnamon essential oil
3 drops rosewood essential oil

In a glass bowl or measuring cup mix the soap, rosewater, and sweet almond oil. Cover and let sit overnight. Add the oatmeal and mix well. Place the mixture in a food processor and mix thoroughly. Add the essential oils one drop at a time, mixing well after each addition. Wet your hands and form the soap into balls, using approximately ½ cup of the mixture at a time. Place them on waxed paper until they are dry and firm.

HERBAL SOAP

1 4-ounce bar of castile soap, grated
3 Tbsp. strong herbal infusion (See directions below.)
1 tsp. ground dried herb, optional (See Suggestions and Variations
    for possible choices.)
4 drops essential oil (See Suggestions and Variations for possible
    choices.)

In a glass bowl or measuring cup mix the herbal infusion and the soap. Cover and let sit overnight. Place the mixture in a food processor and mix. Add the ground dried herb now if desired. Add the essential oil one drop at a time, mixing after each addition. Wet your hands and form the soap into balls using approximately ½ cup of the mixture for each one. Place the soapballs on waxed paper until dry and firm.

To make a strong herbal infusion: Take ¼ cup of dried herb or ½ cup of fresh herb and add to 1 cup of boiling water. Cover the infusion with a saucer or small plate to prevent the herb's essential oils from evaporating. Allow the infusion to steep for 15-20 minutes. Strain the infusion and use in the recipe as directed.

Suggestion and Variations:

- thyme infusion and orange essential oil, optional dried ground thyme leaves

- lavender infusion and rose essential oil, optional dried ground lavender buds

- rosemary infusion and lemon essential oil, optional dried ground rosemary leaves

- calendula infusion and German chamomile essential oil, optional dried ground German chamomile blossoms

- lemon balm infusion and peppermint essential oil, optional dried ground lemon balm leaves

DEODORANT SOAP

This recipe calls for using a soap mold, but you can form the mixture into soap balls if you don't have a mold. Follow the directions from any of the other recipes for molding soapballs.

> ¾ cup rebatchable soap or soap curls
> 1 Tbsp. distilled water
> ½ tsp. baking soda
> 6 drops bergamot essential oil
> soap mold 1 inch deep, 2 inches wide, and 3 inches long
> non stick cooking spray or oil

Spray the soap mold with non-stick cooking spray or wipe a thin coat of oil on the inside surface and set aside. In a heat proof glass container add the soap and distilled water. Place the container in a saucepan with 2 inches of boiling water in it. Heat the mixture, stirring occasionally until it is soft and "mushy". (This takes approximately 25 minutes.) Remove from heat, and stir in the baking soda and essential oil. Using a spatula, place the mixture into the soap mold, pressing it in gently to avoid air spaces and smoothing the top when finished. Allow the soap mixture to cool and dry in the mold. (This takes several hours or overnight.) Remove the soap from the mold, wrap and store as usual.

Variations: Substitute any essential oil of your choice for the bergamot oil. Omit the baking soda and add 1 tsp. dried ground herbs of your choice, dried ground cinnamon, cornmeal, or ground oatmeal.

CUSTOMIZED LIQUID SOAP

Liquid castile soap can be purchased at health food stores. My favorite brand is Dr. Bronner's Aloe Vera Baby Mild Pure Castile Soap. *It is unscented and can be customized as desired.*

> ½ **cup unscented liquid castile soap**
> **6 drops essential oil, your choice**

Mix the essential oil into the liquid soap. Place the soap in a squeeze bottle or small bottle. Use as you would any liquid body soap.

SILKY SMOOTH LIQUID SOAP

The addition of Super Silk to this recipe helps to increase the lathering ability of the soap and gives your skin a smooth feeling.

> ½ **cup unscented liquid castile soap or other unscented liquid soap**
> ⅛ **tsp. Super Silk**
> **8 drops tangerine essential oil**
> **6 drops rosemary essential oil**

Mix all of the ingredients together and place in a squeeze bottle.

Variations: Change the essential oils to your needs and liking, not exceeding 14 drops of essential oil for the recipe.

Body and
Bath Oil

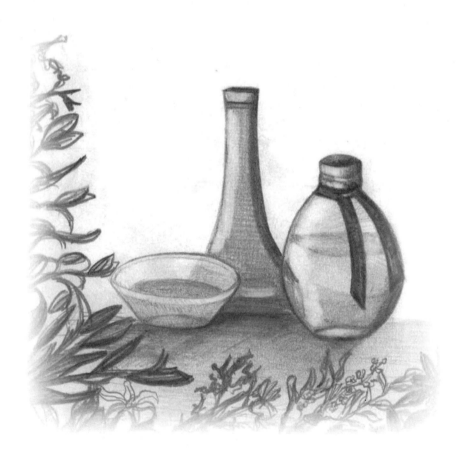

$\mathcal{O}$ have another anecdote to provide proof that you should make your own products! In a popular discount store I saw very small bottles of artificially scented bath oil with dried flowers floating in it for $4 a bottle. I know that you can make a superior quality bath oil for much less than that.

OIL AND WATER DON'T MIX

Due to the nature of their composition, bath oil products float on top of your bath water. This accomplishes two things. It coats your body with the bath oil as you get out of the tub. It also coats the surface of the tub as you drain the water. This creates a hazardous slippery condition that can cause you or the next person who uses the tub to slip and possibly fall.

Essential oils in their pure form will also float on water. You can smell them as you are bathing, but you will receive little of their therapeutic properties on your skin unless they are mixed with another substance such as sea salt, dried milk, oatmeal, or borax. Using essential oils undiluted in the bath also has the potential of adverse reactions to your skin if it comes into contact with the undiluted oils. (See the Bath Time section of this book for more information and recipes.)

Turkey Red Oil is a specially treated oil that will disperse in water. If you want a skin softening bath, this is a good ingredient to use. (Please see Question and Answer section for more information.)

Recommendations for Using Bath Oils:

As your tub is filling with water, massage the bath or body oil into your skin, then soak in the tub as usual. The warmth of the bath water will open your skin pores and allow the oil to work its moisturizing magic.

OR

After drying yourself off from your bath, massage the bath or body oil into your skin.

WORK-WEARY HANDS OIL

Provides heavy duty help and protection to hands that are exposed to cold wet conditions. The essential oil content of this recipe can promote healing for chapped irritated hands. It can also be used as a body oil.

1 Tbsp. castor oil
1 tsp. avocado oil
10 drops evening primrose oil
400 IU Vitamin E
3 drops tea tree essential oil
3 drops German chamomile essential oil

Mix all of the ingredients together. Store in a small glass bottle. Shake well before using.

BEST-EVER BODY OIL

When giving lectures or classes I am frequently asked which recipes are my favorites. This is my number one choice. I use it on a daily basis.

1 Tbsp. avocado oil
20 drops jojoba oil
800 IU Vitamin E
15 drops carrot seed essential oil
8 drops geranium essential oil
2 drops lemon essential oil
2 drops German chamomile essential oil
2 drops sandalwood essential oil

Mix all of the ingredients together. Store in a small glass bottle. Shake well before using.

EXTRA RICH OIL

This blend of several oils can be used on the hands or body.

1 tsp. avocado oil
1 tsp. apricot kernel oil
¼ tsp. jojoba oil
¼ tsp. rosehip seed oil
¼ tsp. wheat germ oil
¼ tsp. castor oil
800 IU Vitamin E
6 drops ylang ylang essential oil
4 drops lavender essential oil
1 drop cinnamon essential oil

Mix all of the ingredients together. Store in a small glass bottle. Shake well before using.

HELPFUL HEALING HAND OIL

The calendula infused oil adds a healing touch to this all purpose oil.

1 Tbsp. calendula infused herbal oil (See the recipe for Infused Oil
   in this section of the book.)
1 tsp. avocado oil
800 IU Vitamin E
6 drops lemon essential oil
4 drops carrot seed essential oil
2 drops frankincense essential oil
2 drops palmarosa essential oil

Mix all of the ingredients together. Store in a small glass bottle. Shake well before using.

CUSTOMIZED DISPERSIBLE BATH OIL

Turkey red oil is water-dispersible, enabling the oil to soak into your skin while you're soaking in the tub.

2 Tbsp. turkey red oil
2-4 drops essential oil, your choice

Mix the ingredients together, then add to your bath water. Bathe as usual.

DISPERSIBLE ROSEWATER BATH OIL

Rosewater adds a floral scent and enhances the softening capability of the turkey red oil.

2 Tbsp. turkey red oil
1 Tbsp. rosewater

Mix the ingredients together, then add to your bath water. Bathe as usual.

NONDISPERSIBLE BATH OIL

This recipe can also be used as a massage oil.

> 1 Tbsp. base oil (sweet almond, apricot kernel, grapeseed, olive, or avocado, your choice)
> 6 drops essential oil, your choice (See the suggestions below for essential oils for massage.)
> 800 IU Vitamin E (Add if the mixture will be kept for more than one use.)

Mix all of the ingredients together. Use immediately after your bath. If there are leftovers, store in a small bottle.

Essential oil additions for the purpose of massage: Keep the total essential oil ratio at 6 drops to every tablespoon of carrier oil.

- For relaxing muscles: lavender, geranium

- For calming and soothing the nerves and spirit: lavender, German chamomile

- For a sore muscle rub or foot massage: rosemary

- For sensual massage: jasmine, rose, sandalwood, ylang ylang

ALL-PURPOSE BODY OIL

Use before or after your bath, or as a massage oil.

> 1 tsp. wheat germ oil
> 1 tsp. avocado oil
> 1 tsp. rosehip seed oil
> 400 IU Vitamin E
> 6 drops essential oil, your choice

Mix all of the ingredients together. Store in a small bottle.

HERBAL INFUSED OIL

This is an ideal way to transfer the properties of any given herb into oil. Olive oil is the best choice for this recipe because it has better keeping qualities than some of the other vegetable oils. Use only dried herbs for any of these infused oil recipes. Fresh herbs have a high water content that can promote mold growth. This oil is for external use only. The internal consumption of herbal infused oils using the recipes in this book is not recommended.

Method no. 1

Fill a glass jar with a tight-fitting lid with the dried herb of your choice. Fill the jar to the top with olive oil. Close the jar and place it in a sunny window for about 2 weeks. Strain the herbs from the oil after the two week period of time. Add 800 IU Vitamin E to the oil as a preservative. Place the infused oil in a glass bottle and label. For extended shelf life, store the oil in the refrigerator.

Method no. 2

> ½ **cup olive oil**
> ¼ **cup dried herb**

In a saucepan, add the ingredients and place on low heat on the stove. Allow the mixture to warm very gently for about 30 minutes. Stir it frequently as it heats. Watch it very carefully. The oil must not be allowed to get so hot that it smokes or spatters. (If it does, it must be discarded and the process started over again.)

After 30 minutes, strain the herbs from the oil and discard. Add 800 IU Vitamin E to the infused oil. Place the infused oil in a glass bottle and label. For an extended shelf life, store the oil in the refrigerator.

Method no. 3

> 1 cup olive oil
> ½ cup dried herb

Mix the ingredients in a slow cooker appliance. Turn the heat setting to its lowest number and put the cover on. Let the oil and dried herbs warm for 4 hours. Strain the herbs from the oil and discard. Add 800 IU Vitamin E to the infused oil Place the infused oil in a glass bottle and label. For an extended shelf life, store the oil in the refrigerator.

"BABY" OIL

Appropriate to use on baby's tender skin as well as on yours!

> 3 Tbsp. jojoba oil
> 1 tsp. evening primrose oil
> 800 IU Vitamin E
> 1 drop German chamomile essential oil
> 1 drop lavender essential oil

Mix all of the ingredients together. Store in a small glass bottle.

PERFUME OIL

Jojoba oil is an ideal carrier for essential oils. Custom blend any combination of essential oils that seems pleasing to you.

> 2 Tbsp. jojoba oil
> 20 drops (more or less) essential oil blends, your choice

Mix the ingredients together. Store in a glass bottle. To use, massage a drop or two on your pulse points where you want fragrance.

Essential oil blend suggestions:

EXOTIC: 10 drops neroli essential oil, 6 drops ylang ylang essential oil, 4 drops frankincense essential oil

FLORAL: 10 drops lavender essential oil, 7 drops rose essential oil, 3 drops patchouli essential oil

LIGHT CITRUS: 12 drops neroli essential oil, 6 drops orange essential oil, 2 drops cinnamon essential oil

BLENDING GUIDE FOR ESSENTIAL OILS

As a beginning, use only 3 different essential oils in a blend. As you become more experienced you can add more. Add only 1 drop at a time and take a light whiff of your blend. Too intense of a scent can be overpowering. Blends generally consist of blending aroma "notes". Here is an further explanation of aroma notes.

Top Notes: *These are scents that are sharp and short. You notice them first when smelling a blend of aromas. EXAMPLES: bergamot, orange, lemon, lime, tangerine, grapefruit, neroli, basil, peppermint, lavender, German chamomile*

Middle Notes: *These scents smooth out the blend. EXAMPLES: rose, geranium ylang ylang, clove, ginger, jasmine*

Base Notes: *These scents add fullness and last longest. They can be deep and earthy. Use these in the smallest amounts in your blend. EXAMPLES: patchouli, sandalwood, frankincense, myrrh, cedarwood, cinnamon*

JASMINE BODY BALM BAR

This unique form of skin care can be rubbed on your skin immediately after a bath or shower to moisturize in a most fragrant way. It can be used any time of the day for areas of your skin that need extra moisturizing.

1½ Tbsp. olive oil
1 Tbsp. beeswax (pearls or solid beeswax grated and measured)
1 tsp. jasmine floral wax
1 tsp. jojoba oil
½ tsp. shea butter
6 drops Super Silk
3 drops tangerine essential oil

Take a clean 8 ounce yogurt cup and cut the sides down until the cup is about 2 inches tall and set aside. Place all of the ingredients except for the Super Silk and essential oil in a heat proof container and melt over boiling water. When the mixture has melted remove it from the heat source. Add the Super Silk and essential oil and mix well. Pour the mixture into the prepared yogurt cup. After the bar has cooled and is solid, pop it out of the yogurt cup. To use, rub on any parts of the skin where you want a moisturizing effect. To store, wrap in plastic wrap or place in a closed container. For portability, the melted mixture could be poured into "push up" containers such as those designed for the use of lip balm.

Facial Care

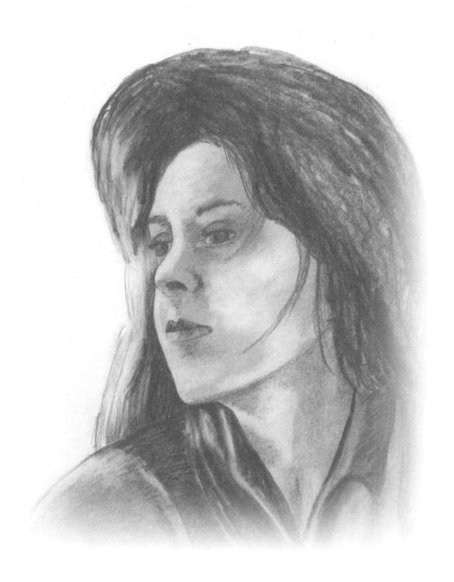

*B*asic skin types are dry, normal, oily, sensitive, and blemished or troubled. Evaluate the type of skin your face has before using any products. You may find that your face has a combination of skin types. This is not uncommon. Simply treat each part of your skin with the appropriate product. When applying any facial product, do so with clean hands to prevent the introduction of any unwanted bacteria.

TIPS FOR SKIN TYPES

Sensitive skin – *Avoid products that can irritate or damage delicate skin such as facial scrubs. Use caution when putting any new product on sensitive skin. The nature of sensitive skin makes it prone to adverse reactions to any number of products or ingredients.*

Oily and/or blemished skin – *Avoid products that are extremely drying – contrary to popular belief, these products can encourage oil production, only making oily skin conditions worse.*

Wrinkled, aging skin – *There are no miracle products that make wrinkles permanently disappear. Some preparations can help to prevent more wrinkles from developing.*

Skin with small broken capillaries – *Treat skin that is prone to this condition with special gentle care. Avoid scrubs and facial steams.*

Skin with rashes or sunburns – *Avoid scrubs or other potentially damaging or irritating treatments. Gentle care is indicated for these conditions.*

Blemished skin – *Handle blemishes with a gentle touch. Don't pick, squeeze, or otherwise try to force blemishes to open and drain. Permanent disfiguring scarring can result from such rough handling.*

HERBAL CLEANSING GRAINS

These grains are a fragrant way to deep-clean normal, oily, and/or blemished skin.

¼ cup cornmeal
¼ cup ground oatmeal
½ cup green clay
1 Tbsp. ground and sifted dried lavender buds
2 Tbsp. finely ground raw sunflower seeds
3 drops lavender essential oil
1 drop patchouli essential oil

Place all of the ingredients except the essential oils in a food processor. Process until the ingredients are uniformly coarse. Add the essential oils and mix well. To use, mix 1-2 tsp. of the mixture with water to form a paste. Gently massage the mixture onto your skin, then rinse well. Pat, don't rub, the skin dry.

FACIAL SCRUB

This mixture can be used on normal, oily, and/or blemished skin.

1 Tbsp. finely ground oatmeal
1 Tbsp. ground and sifted dried lavender buds
1 Tbsp. ground dried thyme leaves
1 Tbsp. finely ground almonds
4 drops lemon essential oil

Mix all of the ingredients except for the essential oil together. Add the essential oil and mix well. To use, mix 1-2 tsp. with enough water to make a paste. Gently massage the mixture onto your skin, then rinse well. Pat, don't rub, the skin dry.

HERB OATMEAL SCRUB

Besides using as a facial scrub, this could be used as an invigorating body scrub during a shower.

> 2 tsp. grated pure soap or castile soap
> 2 tsp. coarsely ground dried rosemary leaves
> 1 tsp. ground oatmeal

Mix all of the ingredients together, and store in a tightly covered jar. To use, place about 1 tsp. onto your wet hand and rub onto your face gently using circular motions. Rinse with cool water and pat dry.

Variations: Substitute coarsely ground dried thyme leaves, ground dried mint leaves, OR ground dried lavender buds for the rosemary.

CUSTOMIZED CLEANSING LOTION

Good for any skin type except dry or sensitive. This can be used as a toner after cleansing your face, or as a middle of the day product for a quick refreshing cleanse.

> ¼ cup distilled water
> 1 Tbsp. rubbing alcohol
> 2½ tsp. witch hazel extract
> 8 drops of lemon, juniper OR lavender essential oils

Add the essential oil of your choice to the alcohol and stir well. Add the rest of the ingredients. Store in a bottle. Shake well before using. To use, apply to cotton pads and gently wipe the face.

DRY SKIN CONDITIONER

The olive oil moisturizes, the honey hydrates, and the vinegar helps to maintain the acid mantle!

> **2 tsp. apple cider vinegar**
> **1 tsp. olive oil**
> **1 tsp. honey**

Mix all of the ingredients together. Apply to your face and leave on for 10-15 minutes. Rinse off with tepid water. Gently pat the face dry. You may finish by applying rosewater to your skin if desired.

OILY FACE RINSE

Oily skin types are prone to blemishes. The herbs in this rinse contain antibacterial properties to help prevent break-outs.

> **1 cup distilled water**
> **1 Tbsp. dried thyme leaves**
> **1 Tbsp dried calendula blossoms**

Put all of the ingredients in a saucepan. Bring to a boil and simmer the mixture covered for 10 minutes. Strain the herbs from the infusion. Allow the infusion to cool to room temperature before using. To use, apply to clean skin and allow to air dry. Leftover infusion can be stored in the refrigerator and used for up to three days.

HERBAL FACIAL RINSE

Pick an herb from the list that best suits your skin type.

2 cups distilled water
¼ cup dried herbs OR ½ cup fresh herbs

In a saucepan bring the distilled water to a boil. Pour the boiling water over the herbs and cover, allowing the mixture to steep for 15-20 minutes. Strain the herbs from the infusion. Allow the infusion to cool to room temperature. Bottle the infusion and store in the refrigerator for up to three days. To use, apply to clean skin and allow to air dry.

Herb choices for different skin types:

- OILY SKIN: rosemary, sage, or yarrow

- NORMAL SKIN: lady's mantle

- DRY SKIN: parsley or lemon balm

- BLEMISHED OR TROUBLED SKIN: chamomile, calendula, rosemary, or thyme

- ALL SKIN TYPES: basil, lavender, mint

- MATURE SKIN: fennel seed or parsley

LAVENDER SKIN FRESHENER

This is a refreshing application for your face and a good middle-of-the-day product. It can be used with all skin types, although for dry skin the applications should be in moderation.

2 Tbsp. distilled water
1 Tbsp. witch hazel extract
1 Tbsp. rosewater
1 drop lavender essential oil

Add the essential oil to the witch hazel extract. Add the rosewater and distilled water. Store in a bottle. Shake well before using. To use, apply with cotton pads.

BRACING ASTRINGENT

This is only for use with oily skin types.

½ **cup distilled water**
⅓ **cup pure grain alcohol or good quality vodka**
¼ **cup dried yarrow**

Mix the yarrow with the alcohol. Let the covered mixture sit for two days. Strain and discard the herbs. Add the distilled water. Store in a bottle. To use, apply with a cotton pad.

TONERS OR ASTRINGENTS?

Toners and astringents are basically the same type of product. They temporarily close your skin pores and leave your skin feeling tight and refreshed. A frequently used ingredient is alcohol which tones or tightens your skin pores. Toners or astringents can dry your skin, so their use is limited to oily, blemished, or normal skin types.

ROSEWATER-LEMON TONER

Lemon juice and rosewater can have softening effects on the skin. This product could be used as an aftershave as well. Use on oily, blemished, or normal skin.

> 3 Tbsp. rosewater
> 2 Tbsp. fresh squeezed and strained lemon juice
> 2 Tbsp. distilled water
> 2 tsp. rubbing alcohol
> 2 drops rosemary essential oil

Mix all of the ingredients together. Place in a bottle. This mixture must be stored in the refrigerator and used within two weeks. Shake before using. To use, apply with a cotton pad.

MULTIPURPOSE FACIAL CARE

This can be used as an aftershave, cleanser, and/or toner. It can also be used as an after-bath body splash. The properties of dried herbs transfer beautifully to the vinegar. This is useful for any skin type.

> 1 cup apple cider vinegar
> ½ cup distilled water
> ½ cup dried herb, your choice

Method no. 1

Place the dried herb in a clean glass jar with a tight fitting lid. Add the vinegar to the jar. Place the lid on the jar and place it in a sunny window for 2 weeks. Strain and discard the herb. Add the distilled water to the herbal vinegar. Store in a bottle away from direct heat and light.

Method no. 2

Place the dried herb and vinegar in a saucepan. Heat over low heat and simmer covered for 30 minutes. Strain and discard the herb. Allow the vinegar to cool to room temperature, then add the distilled water. Store in a bottle away from direct heat and light.

To use, pat or splash the mixture onto your skin, allowing it to air dry.

Suggestions for herbs: lavender, lemon balm, German chamomile, thyme, calendula, rosemary

ROSEWATER ASTRINGENT

This recipe is appropriate for normal or oily skin.

> 3 tsp. rosewater
> 1 tsp. witch hazel extract
> 1 tsp. apple cider vinegar
> 1 drop orange essential oil
> 1 drop juniper essential oil

Mix all of the ingredients together. Store in a bottle. To use, splash on or apply with cotton pads.

Variation: Substitute one drop of cedarwood essential oil and one drop rosemary essential oil for the orange and juniper essential oils. The woodsy scent makes it appropriate for use as an aftershave.

OILY SKIN FRESHENER

It smells fresh, is simple to make, and makes your skin feel clean and soft. What more could you want?

> **1 Tbsp. strained fresh lemon juice**
> **1 Tbsp. distilled water**

Mix together and apply with cotton pads.

FACIAL SPRITZER, 2 WAYS

Use these recipes as facial or overall skin refreshers. It is especially refreshing when used during hot humid weather.

First Way:

> **2 cups distilled water**
> **¼ cup pure grain alcohol or good quality vodka**
> **10 drops essential oil, your choice**

Mix the alcohol and essential oil together. Let sit for 30 minutes, then add the distilled water. Place the mixture in a spray bottle. Shake before using. Close your eyes before spraying on your face.

Essential oil suggestions:

- 8 drops lavender essential oil, 2 drops peppermint essential oil

- 6 drops rose essential oil, 4 drops lemon essential oil

- 6 drops neroli essential oil, 4 drops lemon essential oil

- 8 drops rosemary essential oil, 2 drops orange essential oil

Second Way:

> 2 cups distilled water
> 1 cup dried lavender buds, dried mint leaves (your choice), dried
>   rosemary leaves, OR dried lemon balm leaves
> ¼ cup pure grain alcohol or good quality vodka

In a saucepan, combine the dried herbs and distilled water. Bring to a boil, then simmer covered for 15 minutes over low heat. Remove from heat, cover, and let the mixture sit for 30 minutes. Strain the herbs from the infusion and discard. Add the alcohol to the infusion. Place the mixture in a spray bottle. Shake before using. Close your eyes before spraying on your face.

TONING ESSENTIAL OILS

The following essential oils have toning qualities and can be substituted in equal amounts for any of the essential oils in toner recipes.

basil	lemon	pine
frankincense	lime	rose
cypress	myrrh	rosemary
jasmine	neroli	tangerine
juniper	orange	thyme
lavender	peppermint	

FACIAL SPRITZER, YOUR WAY

¾ cup distilled water

1 Tbsp. witch hazel extract

5 drops essential oil, your choice (You may use one essential oil or a
blend of more than one.)

Mix the essential oil and the witch hazel extract. Let it sit for 30 minutes,
then add the distilled water. Place in a spray bottle. Shake well before
using. Close your eyes before spraying it on your face.

JOJOBA FACIAL OIL

Apply this to normal, dry, or aging skin for a protective moisturizing coating.

1 Tbsp. jojoba oil

3 drops carrot seed essential oil

3 drops lavender essential oil

2 drops geranium essential oil

Mix all of the ingredients together. Store in a dark glass bottle. Shake well
before using. Massage a small amount into your clean face. If there is any
excess, wipe it off with a tissue or cotton pad.

OILY SKIN FACIAL OIL

Yes, even oily skin can have a moisturizing oil applied to it. This is especially beneficial in the winter months when cold air takes the moisture out of your skin. The specific essential oils in this recipe have cleansing qualities. It won't make your skin feel too greasy or oily. Use it only once a day.

> 1 Tbsp. apricot kernel oil
> 400 IU Vitamin E
> 3 drops juniper essential oil
> 1 drop lemon essential oil
> 1 drop bergamot essential oil

Mix all of the ingredients together. Store the mixture in a small bottle. Shake well before using. Massage a small amount into your clean face. If there is any excess, wipe it off with a tissue or cotton pad.

DRY SKIN FACIAL OIL

Use this after a bath or shower when your skin is moist and/or at night after facial cleansing. It is good for dry or mature skin.

> 1 Tbsp. sweet almond oil
> 2 tsp. avocado oil
> ¼ tsp. rosehip seed oil
> 800 IU Vitamin E
> 5 drops carrot seed essential oil
> 2 drops sandalwood essential oil
> 1 drop myrrh essential oil

Mix all of the ingredients together. Store the mixture in a small bottle. Shake well before using. Massage a small amount into your clean face. If there is any excess, wipe it off with a tissue or cotton pad.

OILY SKIN NIGHT GEL

This mixture will moisturize your skin while you sleep, leaving it feeling clean and non-greasy,.

> 1 Tbsp. aloe vera gel
> 1 tsp. witch hazel extract
> 1 tsp. evening primrose oil
> 2 drops lavender essential oil
> 1 drop lemon essential oil

After facial cleansing, gently massage a small amount onto the skin of your face. Leave it on overnight.

Variation:

Substitute 1 drop of tea tree oil for the lemon essential oil if you are prone to skin blemishes.

ALOE CLEANSING GEL

A perfect cleanser to use before applying any other facial care products.

> ¼ cup aloe vera gel
> 1 Tbsp. grated pure soap
> 2 drops essential oil, your choice

Mix all the ingredients together in a small bowl. Let the mixture sit overnight to let the aloe vera gel soften the grated soap. Stir gently. Store in a small bottle or wide mouth jar. To use, place 1-2 tsp. of the mixture in your hands, add water and work into a lather, and cleanse as usual.

Suggestion: The lather from this gel makes a good shaving cream for men or women.

BLEMISHED SKIN COMPRESSES

An alternative to a facial steam, these compresses open skin pores and allow the beneficial properties of the herbs to work.

> **1 quart water**
> **½ cup dried rosemary leaves**
> **½ cup dried calendula blossoms**

In a saucepan bring the quart of water to a boil. Remove from the heat and add the herbs. Cover the pan and steep the mixture for 20 minutes. Strain the herbs and discard. Let the infusion cool to warm. You should be able to put your hand in the infusion and keep it there for several minutes without pulling it back because it feels too hot. Soak a clean washcloth with the infusion and wring the excess from it. With your eyes closed, place the washcloth on your face for 15 minutes. Remove the washcloth from your face and apply a toner or astringent.

Variation: Substitute 1 cup dried thyme leaves for the rosemary and calendula. Follow the same directions.

ALOE MAKEUP REMOVER

> **1 tsp. aloe vera gel**
> **1 tsp. jojoba oil**

Mix the two ingredients together. Gently apply to your face. Use cotton pads or tissues to wipe off the makeup and remover.

Face Masks

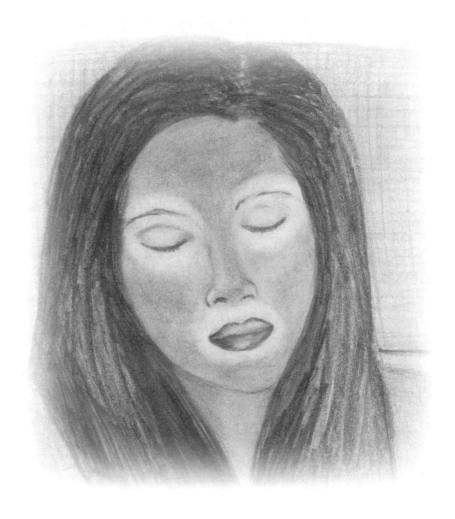

$\mathcal{F}$ace masks can be made from a variety of materials depending on what type of skin you have. Each of these recipes will make note of what skin type can appropriately use each mask.

FACE MASK PRIMER

⚘ *Always cleanse your face before applying a face mask.*

⚘ *Face masks containing clay will draw oils and impurities from your skin.*

⚘ *Face masks containing oils, brewer's yeast, or oatmeal will provide nourishment to your skin.*

⚘ *For dry skin types, clay masks may be used if a thin layer of sweet almond, grapeseed, or apricot kernel oil is applied to the skin first. Do not remove the oil, but apply the clay mask over it and use as directed.*

⚘ *Skin frequently is reddened after using a face mask. Do not apply one immediately prior to going out.*

⚘ *Remove face masks by rinsing with cool water and rubbing gently if needed. Pat your face dry with a soft towel—do not rub the skin hard.*

⚘ *Immediately following a face mask application, apply a toner or astringent if desired.*

⚘ *CAUTION: A burning feeling on your skin while wearing a face mask can signal an adverse reaction to the application. Remove the mask immediately should this sensation occur, and repeatedly rinse your face with cool water.*

LEMON MASK

Use this mask on oily skin. As it dries it feels quite tight. Your skin will feel quite smooth after using this.

1 Tbsp. green clay
1-2 Tbsp. strained lemon juice

In a small bowl, mix the lemon juice into the clay. The mixture will appear foamy and can easily be smoothed onto your skin. Leave on for 20 minutes or until dry. Rinse off with cool or tepid water. Pat your face dry.

JOJOBA MASK

This one is for oily skin.

1 Tbsp. green clay
5 drops jojoba oil
2 drops lavender essential oil

Mix the above ingredients together, then add enough water to make a paste that spreads easily. Smooth onto your face and leave on for 20 minutes or until dry. Rinse off with cool or tepid water. Pat your face dry.

BREWER'S YEAST MASK

Brewer's yeast is soothing and adds nutrients to the skin. This is good for normal to oily and/or troubled skin.

1 Tbsp. brewer's yeast
2 tsp. witch hazel extract
1 drop German chamomile essential oil

Mix all of the ingredients together and add enough water to make a paste that spreads easily. Smooth the mixture onto your face. It will be a bit lumpy. Leave on for 15 minutes, then rinse off with cool or tepid water. Pat your face dry.

SMOOTHING MASK

Flaxseeds form a gel when soaked or boiled in water. The gel does not feel overly tight while it is drying. This is good for any skin type.

2 tsp. flaxseeds
water-enough to cover

In a small bowl, mix the water and flaxseeds. Let it sit until the seeds swell and the water turns to gel. Spread the gel on your face using your fingers. Allow to dry, then rinse off with cool or tepid water. Pat your face dry.

Variations: If desired, mix **one drop** of any of the following essential oils to the flaxseed gel before applying it to your face according to your skin's needs.

- OILY SKIN: cedarwood, peppermint, rose

- MATURE AND/OR WRINKLED SKIN: frankincense, neroli

- NORMAL SKIN: lavender, ylang ylang

- SENSITIVE SKIN: jasmine, rose, German chamomile

- DRY SKIN: carrot seed, sandalwood

MATURE OR DRY SKIN MASK

The skin on your face will feel soft and smell good after using this mask!

1 Tbsp. brewer's yeast
1 tsp. crushed fennel seeds
½ cup water

In a small saucepan simmer the fennel seeds in water for 10 minutes and strain. (Do not keep the fennel seeds in the water any longer than 10 minutes or they will soak up all of the infusion.) Let the infusion cool to room temperature, then mix in the brewer's yeast. Spread the mixture on your face and leave on for 10 minutes. Rinse off with cool or tepid water. Pat your face dry.

CLAY MASK

This mask is appropriate for use on oily skin.

> **1 Tbsp. fuller's earth**
> **1 drop lavender essential oil**

Add the essential oil to the fuller's earth and stir. Add enough water to the mixture to make a paste that spreads easily. Smooth the mixture on your face and leave on for 20 minutes or until dry. Rinse off with cool or tepid water. Pat your face dry.

Variation: For blemished skin, substitute 1 drop of tea tree essential oil for the lavender essential oil. Use as directed.

WONDERFUL CLAY

Any of the available cosmetic clays will absorb moisture and oil when applied to any part of the body. They will also draw impurities from your skin and body. Best of all, they are some of the most inexpensive ingredients around!

LADY'S MANTLE MASK

Lady's mantle is an herb that is a natural astringent. This mask can be used on normal to oily skin.

> **1 Tbsp. brewer's yeast**
> **2 tsp. rosewater**
> **1 Tbsp. dried lady's mantle leaves**
> **⅔ cup boiling water**

Pour the boiling water over the dried lady's mantle leaves. Let the mixture steep for 10 minutes. Strain the herb from the infusion and set aside. Reserve 1 Tbsp. of the infusion for use in the mask. (The remainder of the infusion can be refrigerated for up to three days and used as an astringent facial rinse if desired.) Mix the brewer's yeast, rosewater, and herbal infusion together. Smooth the mixture onto your face and leave on for 15 minutes. Rinse off with cool or tepid water. Pat your face dry.

FENNEL SEED MASK

The mixture of fennel and oatmeal is soothing and would be appropriate for dry, sensitive, and/or mature skin.

> 1 Tbsp. honey
> 1 Tbsp. ground oatmeal
> 2 tsp. crushed fennel seeds
> ⅓ cup boiling water

Add the crushed fennel seeds to the boiling water. Let the mixture infuse for 15 minutes, then strain and discard the seeds. Reserve 1 Tbsp. of the infusion for the recipe. (The remaining infusion can be refrigerated and used within three days as a facial rinse.) Mix the 1 Tbsp. fennel seed infusion and the honey. Add the oatmeal and mix well. Smooth the mixture on your face. Leave on for 15 minutes, then rinse with cool or tepid water. Pat your skin dry.

OATMEAL MASK

Oatmeal is beneficial for any skin type.

> 1 Tbsp. ground oatmeal
> rosewater

Add rosewater by the teaspoonful to the oatmeal until the mixture can be easily spread. Smooth the mixture onto your face and leave on until it is dry. Rinse off with cool or tepid water. Pat your skin dry.

OATMEAL HERBAL FACE TREATMENT

Oatmeal is good for any skin type. Choose an herb that suits your skin's needs.

1 Tbsp. ground oatmeal
3 Tbsp. dried herb, your choice
⅔ cup boiling water

Make the herbal infusion by pouring the boiling water over the dried herb. Allow the infusion to steep covered for 15 minutes. Strain and discard the herb. Let the infusion cool to room temperature. Add enough of the infusion to the oatmeal to make a consistency that will spread easily. (Save the remaining herbal infusion.) Smooth the mask on your face and leave on for 20 minutes. Rinse off with cool or tepid water and pat your face dry. Use the reserved herbal infusion as a facial lotion after drying your face.

Possible Herb Choices:

- OILY SKIN: sage, yarrow, or lady's mantle

- DRY, AGING SKIN: parsley, lemon balm, or fennel seed

- SENSITIVE SKIN: German chamomile

- BLEMISHED SKIN: thyme, calendula, or rosemary

- ANY SKIN TYPE: lavender, basil, or mint (your choice)

Variation:

Substitute 1 Tbsp. of any clay for the oatmeal. Before applying to dry or aging skin, coat the face with a thin layer of sweet almond, apricot kernel, or grapeseed oil. Follow the rest of the application instructions as outlined above.

NOURISHING FACE MASK

This can be used on any type of skin.

> **1 Tbsp. apple cider vinegar**
> **1 Tbsp. honey**

Mix the two ingredients together and smooth onto your clean face. Leave the mixture on for 15-20 minutes, then rinse off with tepid water. Pat your face dry.

DRY SKIN FACE MASK

Nourishing ingredients supply your skin with moisture.

> **2 Tbsp. avocado oil**
> **1 Tbsp. finely ground oatmeal**
> **400 IU Vitamin E**
> **1 drop carrot seed essential oil**

Mix all of the ingredients together and smooth the mixture onto your clean face. Leave the mixture on for 15-20 minutes, then rinse off with tepid water. Pat your face dry.

Variations: Substitute one drop of jasmine essential oil, geranium essential oil, ylang ylang essential oil, OR rosewood essential oil for the carrot seed essential oil.

After Sun Care

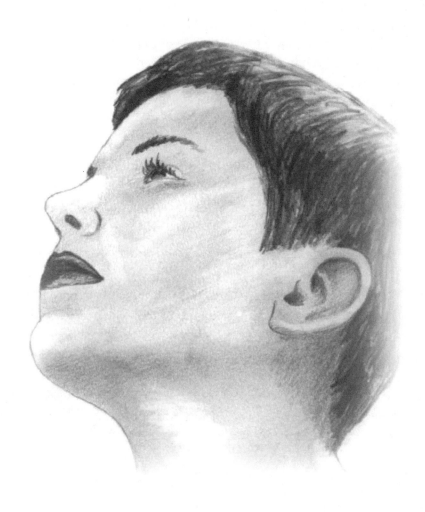

Sunlight and Ultraviolet Rays

Sunlight contains ultraviolet, or UV, rays. The two most common UV rays that are mentioned in connection with adverse effects to the skin are UVA and UVB rays. 90-95% of sunlight consists of UVA rays. These rays penetrate furthest into the skin and can help to contribute to skin damage. UVB rays do not penetrate the skin as deeply as UVA rays. They are the primary cause of sunburns and other tissue damage contributed to overexposure to sunlight.

Sunlight isn't always a "bad guy". Our skin's exposure to sunlight helps our body to manufacture Vitamin D, an important nutrient. Moderate sun exposure at times of the day when the sun isn't at its most intense (before 11 AM or after 2 PM) will give your body the chance to produce Vitamin D without sustaining skin and tissue damage from overexposure to the sun's potentially damaging rays. It is thought that 10-15 minutes of unprotected exposure to sunlight daily is enough for your body to manufacture Vitamin D.

Despite warnings about protecting our skin from the sun, we all know people (ourselves included) who push the limits and come inside with reddened and painful skin. Included here are some recipes to help relieve the discomfort. These are meant to be used only on reddened, not blistered, skin.

NATURAL SUNSCREENS

A few of the vegetable oils listed in this book have very low SPF (Sun Protection Factor). This is the number that is listed on sunscreen bottles with the higher numbers signifying a longer amount of time that the sun's rays are filtered after application of the product. It is my opinion that, due to the difficulty in finding many of the ingredients and specific directions for production, natural sunscreen products are too complicated to make in your kitchen. It is best to purchase a sunscreen and wear it to help avoid damage from overexposure to the sun. When shopping for a sunscreen, look for a product that has vegetable oils or butters as a base rather than mineral oil. For information on the derivation of specific ingredients and their actions, check with the individual manufacturer or do an Internet search typing in the words "natural sunscreen". You will find a wealth of information on the topic. (See the Resources section of this book for information on where to purchase natural sunscreen products.)

SKIN COOLING SUMMER BATH

**¼ cup dried peppermint leaves or ½ cup fresh peppermint leaves
1 cup distilled water**

In a saucepan bring the distilled water to a boil. Add the peppermint and simmer covered for 15 minutes. Strain the herb from the infusion and discard. Allow the infusion to cool to lukewarm. Add the infusion to tepid bathwater and soak for 15-20 minutes.

Variation: Substitute ¼ cup dried German chamomile blossoms for the peppermint leaves.

SUNBURN SOAK

Lavender has healing properties that are ideal for sunburn care.

**1 cup apple cider vinegar
10 drops lavender essential oil**

Mix the two ingredients together. Add to tepid bath water. Soak in the tub and sponge affected skin.

LAVENDER SUNBURN RINSE

1 quart water
1 Tbsp. pure grain alcohol
10 drops lavender essential oil

Add the essential oil to the pure grain alcohol. Let sit for 30 minutes. Add the distilled water. Dip a sponge or soft cloth into the mixture and apply to sunburn or spray on affected areas. Store the remainder in a bottle and label.

HERBAL SUNBURN RINSE

¼ cup dried calendula blossoms
2 cups distilled water

In a saucepan bring the distilled water to a boil. Add the calendula blossoms and simmer covered for 30 minutes. Strain the herbs from the infusion and discard. Allow the infusion to cool. To use, add ¼ cup of the infusion to 1 cup cool water. Dip a sponge or soft cloth into the mixture and apply to sunburn. The infusion may be stored in the refrigerator and used for up to three days.

LAVENDER ALOE RELIEF

Two sunburn relievers are combined to make one cooling combination.

1 Tbsp. aloe vera gel
5 drops lavender essential oil

Mix the two ingredients and apply directly to sunburned areas.

Variation: Substitute lemon essential oil OR German chamomile essential oil for the lavender essential oil.

BODY TEA

The tannins that are present in black tea help to relieve the discomfort from sunburn.

3 black tea bags
1 quart water

In a saucepan bring the water to a boil. Add the tea bags and remove the saucepan from the heat. Let the tea bags steep for 30 minutes. Remove the tea bags from the infusion and discard. Place the infusion in the refrigerator until it is cold. Gently sponge areas that have been sunburned with the infusion. Allow the infusion to air dry on the skin. Leftover tea may be stored in the refrigerator and used within 3-5 days. Discard any leftovers after that period of time.

CAUTION, CAUTION, CAUTION

§ *Some medications can make you more susceptible to sunburn. If you are taking any medicines consult your health care provider and/or your pharmacist for more information.*

§ *Do not expose sunburned skin to more sun. You will only increase the damage that has already occurred.*

§ *Once your skin is reddened, damage has already been sustained. The effects of sun exposure can worsen once you are out of the sun. That is to say, red skin can get redder, and possibly blister.*

§ *Blistered skin indicates second degree burns. These blisters can break, leaving open areas on your body that are susceptible to infection.*

§ *Oils applied to sunburned skin tend to trap the heat and will make you feel more uncomfortable.*

§ *You can be just as prone to sunburn on overcast days. Burning UVA rays can penetrate cloud cover, so take the usual precautions to protect yourself from sunburn.*

- *There is an increased risk of sun damage at higher elevations.*

- *No sunscreen will block 100% of the sun's rays.*

- *Sand, water, pavement, tall buildings, and snow all reflect sunlight, increasing your chances for a sunburn.*

- *The lighter your skin and hair, the more susceptible you are to sunburn.*

- *Seek the advice of a health care professional for unusual skin growths or moles. Be especially alert to any skin growths that are irregularly shaped, bleed easily, itch, and/or change shape or color.*

- *The rays from a tanning booth session have the potential to cause the same damage to your skin as natural sunlight.*

SUNBURN SPRAY

This may be applied several times a day. For extra relief, store this spray in the refrigerator to chill the product before use.

> ¼ cup distilled water
> 2 Tbsp. aloe vera gel
> 1 Tbsp. witch hazel extract
> 6 drops lavender essential oil
> 1 drop German chamomile essential oil
> 1 drop tea tree essential oil

Mix the essential oils with the witch hazel extract. Add the distilled water and the aloe vera gel. Store in a spray bottle. Shake well before using. Spray where desired. Avoid eye contact.

Variation: For extra healing power, substitute calendula infusion for the distilled water. To make the infusion, boil the ¼ cup of distilled water and pour over 2 Tbsp. dried calendula blossoms. Steep covered for 20 minutes. Strain the herbs from the infusion and follow the above instructions to make the Sunburn Spray using the calendula infusion instead of the distilled water.

Natural Beauty Basics

AFTER-SUN SKIN CONDITIONER

This lotion will help to maintain your skin's moisture. It may be used on skin that has been exposed to sunlight without being burned.

½ tsp. sweet almond oil OR rosehip seed oil
½ tsp. aloe vera gel
⅛ tsp. liquid lecithin
12 drops evening primrose oil
1 drop tea tree essential oil
1 drop carrot seed essential oil

Using a whisk, mix the oil of your choice, the evening primrose oil, and the liquid lecithin together. Add the aloe vera gel and mix with a whisk. Add the essential oils and mix again. Gently massage the mixture into your skin. Store any leftovers in a small bottle or jar. Shake or stir before using.

PROTECTIVE EFFECTS OF GREEN TEA

Recent studies have shown that drinking green tea can markedly decrease your chances of skin cancer. Decaffeinated green tea does not seem to have the protective effects that the tea with caffeine has. Precautions to avoid overexposure to sun should still be followed.

Hair Care

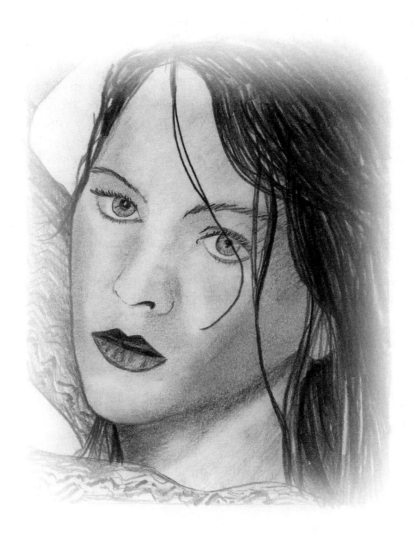

$\mathcal{S}$ome characteristics of your hair are not easily changed. Your hair's texture and degree of oiliness that it normally has are mostly hereditary. Other factors that figure into the condition of your hair are illnesses, inadequate diets, or medications that you are taking.

Hair is composed of dead cells and will not absorb many substances. Commercial hair thickeners coat the hair and make it seem thicker. Oil treatments coat the hair and give it shine. As with other products, read the labels for ingredients on hair care products that are advertised as "natural" or "herbal". You might be surprised to see few herbs or herbal derivatives actually listed on the label.

Try to keep hair care simple. Don't let yourself get bogged down with a bathroom shelf full of products. If you have dry hair, give it an oil treatment and use herbs and essential oils that are appropriate for dry hair. If you have oily hair, use herbs and essential oils to help decrease the oiliness. Want shiny hair? Use lemon juice or apple cider vinegar as a hair rinse. This will give your hair a natural shine.

SCALP TREATMENT FOR DRY HAIR

The skin cells on dry scalp can flake off and shower you and your clothing with unsightly dandruff. Use this treatment once a week to nourish the scalp and help to prevent this from occurring.

> **1 Tbsp. jojoba oil**
> **5 drops carrot seed essential oil**

Mix the two ingredients together. Gently massage your scalp and the shafts of hair coming directly out of your scalp. Wrap you head in a towel, wait one hour, then remove the towel and shampoo as usual.

Variation: For dry brittle hair, substitute 3 drops rosemary essential oil for the carrot seed essential oil. Follow the above directions for use.

OLIVE OIL TREATMENT

This is an appropriate treatment for dry hair and scalp. Use this once a week to help lend a lovely sheen to your hair.

> **1 Tbsp. olive oil**

Gently warm the olive oil in a heat proof container placed in boiling water. The temperature of the olive oil should feel comfortably warm. You should be able to put a finger in the olive oil and be able to keep it there without pulling back because it is too hot. Gently rub the warmed olive oil into your scalp and hair. Wrap your head in a clean, old towel, wait for 20 minutes, then shampoo as usual.

Variation: Substitute rosemary infused oil or lavender infused oil for the olive oil. (See the recipe for Herbal Infused Oil in the Body and Bath Oil section of this book.)

CUSTOMIZED SHAMPOO

This recipe will serve you as well as some of the more expensive shampoos on the market.

> **1 Tbsp. high quality baby shampoo**
> **4 drops essential oil suited to your hair type (See suggestions below.)**

Mix the essential oils of your choice into the shampoo. Apply the shampoo to wet hair, gently rub it into your hair and scalp, and rinse until all trace of the shampoo is gone. Dry and style as usual.

Essential oil suggestions:

- NORMAL HAIR: patchouli, juniper, rosemary, lavender, geranium, OR clary sage

- OILY HAIR: lemon, bergamot, juniper, rosemary, thyme, OR ylang ylang

- DRY HAIR: lavender, carrot seed, sandalwood, OR cedarwood

CONDITIONERS AND HAIR

Use moderation in the frequency of applying conditioning treatments to your hair. Too much conditioning can result in limp hair that seems too oily. If your hair is oily or if you have baby fine hair you are more susceptible to over conditioning.

If you suffer from hair loss due to any variety of causes do not apply a conditioner to your hair. The added weight to the hair shaft can cause an increase in hair loss.

Avoid overconditioning fragile easily breakable hair. The added weight of the conditioner can cause hair to break off, compounding the problem.

CONDITIONING SHAMPOO

D-panthenol is the one vitamin that hair seems to absorb. It strengthens the hair shaft from within and gives your hair a nice shine, too.

> **1 Tbsp. high quality baby shampoo**
> **¼ tsp. d-panthenol**

Mix the two ingredients together, then shampoo your hair as usual.

Variations: Add 4 drops of essential oil of your choice to the above recipe for added benefits to your hair.

SHAMPOO FOR DRY HAIR

1 Tbsp. high quality baby shampoo
5 drops jojoba oil
4 drops carrot seed essential oil

Mix all of the ingredients together, then shampoo your hair as usual.

Variations: Substitute sandalwood essential oil OR cedarwood essential oil for the carrot seed essential oil.

OILY HAIR SHAMPOO

This is my shampoo of choice. I use it on a daily basis.

½ cup high quality baby shampoo
2 Tbsp. aloe vera gel
8 drops rosemary essential oil
2 drops lemon essential oil

Mix all of the ingredients together. Store in a plastic squeeze bottle. To use, squeeze about ½–1 tablespoon of the shampoo onto your hand, apply to wet hair, and shampoo as usual.

MAKING SHAMPOO IN LARGER QUANTITIES

Any of the shampoo recipes may be made in a larger quantity. Keep the proportions of ingredients in any given recipe the same, and place the finished product in a plastic squeeze bottle. Store the bottle near where you are accustomed to shampooing your hair.

DRY HAIR SHAMPOO

¼ cup high quality baby shampoo
2 tsp. sweet almond oil
6 drops sandalwood essential oil

Mix all ingredients together and store in a squeeze bottle. To use, squeeze ½–1 tablespoon onto wet hair and shampoo as usual.

LEMON AFTER-SHAMPOO
HAIR RINSE

This rinse gives your hair shine. Lemon juice is especially beneficial for blonde hair, but other hair colors can use it too.

¼ cup fresh squeezed and strained lemon juice
¼ cup water

Mix together and apply to freshly shampooed hair. Leave on your hair for 10-15 minutes, then rinse with water.

Helpful Hint: Fresh lemons can be squeezed and the juice strained ahead of time. Store this juice in the refrigerator in a covered container. It will keep for a week or two this way and you will have lemon juice available for use whenever you want it for hair or skin care.

VINEGAR AFTER-SHAMPOO RINSE

This can be used on any hair type.

¼ cup apple cider vinegar
¼ cup distilled water

Mix the two ingredients together. After shampooing, rub about half of the mixture into your hair. Leave on for 15 minutes, then rinse with water. Leftovers can be stored in a bottle for future use.

HERBAL HAIR RINSE

Choose an herb that suits your hair color.

2 cups apple cider vinegar
½ cup dried herb of your choice (See list below for suggestions.)

In a saucepan heat the vinegar over low heat and add the herbs to it. Let the mixture simmer covered for about 30 minutes. Remove from the heat. Strain the herbs from the infused vinegar and discard. Allow the vinegar to cool to room temperature. To use, add equal parts of distilled water to the herb infused vinegar. Rub about ½ cup of the vinegar/water mixture into freshly shampooed hair. Leave on your hair for 15 minutes, then rinse with water. The remaining mixture can be stored in a bottle for future use.

Suggested herbs:

- DARK HAIR: rosemary, sage

- LIGHT HAIR: German chamomile

- RED/AUBURN HAIR: calendula

BROWN HAIR RINSE

This infusion will serve to give highlights to brown hair. It won't change your hair color to brown. Highlights will be more noticeable if you use this recipe consistently over a period of time.

> ¼ **cup dried rosemary leaves OR dried sage leaves**
> **2 cups distilled water**

In a saucepan place the two ingredients, cover, and simmer over low heat for 30 minutes. Remove from heat and strain the herbs from the infusion and discard them. Allow the infusion to cool to lukewarm. Over a pan or basin pour the infusion over freshly washed hair. Pour the infusion that was caught in the pan over your hair once again. Dry and style your hair as usual.

Variations:

- LIGHT OR BLONDE HAIR RINSE: Substitute dried German chamomile blossoms for the rosemary or sage. Follow the same basic directions.

- RED OR AUBURN HAIR RINSE: Substitute dried calendula blossoms for the rosemary or sage. Follow the same basic directions.

FRAGRANT HAIR OIL

Hair holds fragrance easily. Take this simple step to give your hair a pleasant aroma.

> **3 drops rosemary essential oil OR**
> **3 drops lavender essential oil**

Midway into drying your hair, place the 3 drops of essential oil of your choice onto your hand. Rub your hands together, then wipe them into your hair. Finish drying and styling your hair as usual.

Variation: For dry hair, add the essential oil to ¼ tsp. of jojoba oil. Massage the mixture into your hair while it is damp, then dry and style your hair as usual.

Natural Beauty Basics

HAIR LOSS

If you are suffering significant hair loss, seek the advice of a health care professional. Certain illnesses can cause hair loss and should be ruled out. Treat your hair and scalp gently if your are suffering from hair loss. Avoid harsh chemicals, exposure to chlorine from swimming pools, and heavy oil and conditioning treatments. Follow a well-balanced diet. Make and use hair care products using your choice of the following essential oils.

cedarwood	*lavender*	*rosemary*
German chamomile	*lemon*	*patchouli*
clary sage	*juniper*	*rose*
cypress	*grapefruit*	*ylang ylang*

SILKY CONDITIONING SHAMPOO

The proteins and amino acids present in the ingredient "Super Silk" help to lend shine without oiliness to any hair type.

> ½ **cup high quality baby shampoo**
> **1 Tbsp. aloe vera gel**
> ⅛ **tsp. Super Silk**
> **10 drops essential oil, your choice (You may use one essential oil or a combination of two.)**

Mix all of the ingredients together. Store in a plastic squeeze bottle. To use, squeeze about ½–1 tablespoon of the shampoo onto your hand, apply to wet hair, and shampoo as usual.

I use a generic baby shampoo for the recipes in this section. Any commercial shampoos that you purchase may have ingredients included that you don't want to use or can't use. If you can't find a baby shampoo that you want to use, you can substitute liquid castile soap in any of these recipes for the baby shampoo in equal amounts. The liquid castile soap may leave a dulling film on your hair. You can restore the shine to your hair by finishing your shampoo with an acidic rinse containing lemon juice or vinegar. Appropriate acidic hair rinse recipes include Lemon After Shampoo Hair Rinse, Vinegar After Shampoo Rinse, or Herbal Hair Rinse, which are included in this section.

Nail Care

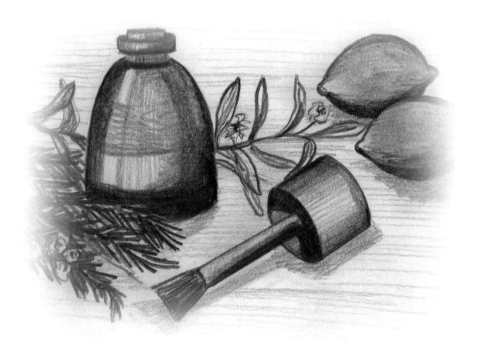

$\mathcal{F}$ingernails and cuticles can get a lot of abuse from housework, gardening, and other activities. Wear gloves when your hands are exposed to harsh conditions to help protect your hands and nails from damage. Some commercial nail hardeners contain formaldehyde which can damage some nails and cuticles due to sensitivity reactions.

NAIL AND CUTICLE OIL

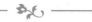

Keeping your cuticles lubricated helps to soften them and prevent the formation of hangnails, a tearing of the cuticles.

½ tsp. sweet almond oil
¼ tsp. jojoba oil
400 IU Vitamin E
2 drops carrot seed essential oil
2 drops lemon essential oil
1 drop eucalyptus essential oil

Mix together and rub a very small amount into nails and cuticles twice a day. Store leftovers in an amber or brown-colored glass bottle.

CITRUS-ROSEMARY NAIL AND CUTICLE OIL

¼ tsp. wheat germ oil
¼ tsp. rosehip seed oil
3 drops grapefruit essential oil
2 drops lemon essential oil
2 drops rosemary essential oil

Mix all ingredients and store in an amber or brown-colored glass bottle. Rub a very small amount into cuticles twice a day.

CUTICLE SOFTENING OIL

¼ tsp. avocado oil
20 drops evening primrose oil
5 drops grapefruit essential oil
5 drops carrot seed essential oil

Mix all ingredients and place in an amber or brown-colored glass bottle. Rub a very small amount into nails and cuticles two or three times a day.

FINGERNAIL OIL

1 tsp. castor oil
400 IU Vitamin E
6 drops lavender essential oil
2 drops sandalwood essential oil

Mix all of the ingredients and place in an amber or brown-colored glass bottle. Before using, shake well. Rub a very small amount into your nails two times a day.

Foot Care

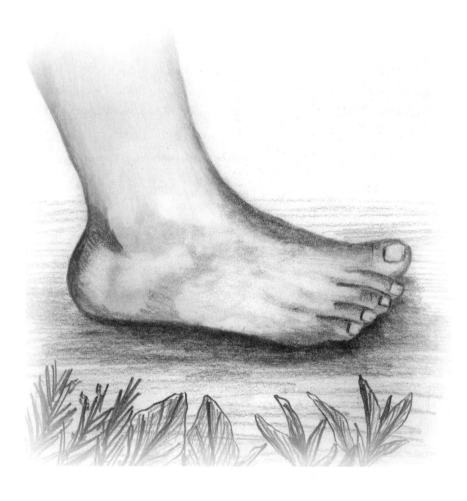

*H*ow many miles do you walk in a year? How about in a week? It is obvious that your feet work hard for you. Take good care of them. Use some of the following recipes to treat your feet.

COOLING FOOT POWDER

This product really helps to keep foot odor and moisture to a minimum.

> ½ **cup arrowroot powder**
> 2 **Tbsp. clay, your choice**
> 1 **tsp. rubbing alcohol**
> 10 **drops peppermint essential oil**
> 8 **drops tea tree essential oil**

Mix all of the ingredients together in a glass container. Cover and let sit for at least 4 hours. Place in a shaker container. Any leftovers can be stored in a glass jar.

Variations: Substitute cypress essential oil OR rosemary essential oil for the tea tree essential oil.

CALLUS TREATMENT

If you don't have any clove essential oil, use the rosehip seed oil by itself. It is very softening on its own. This recipe can also be used on other roughened areas of the skin such as knees and elbows.

> 1 **Tbsp. rosehip seed oil**
> 2 **drops clove essential oil**

Mix the two ingredients together and store in a glass bottle. Rub a very small amount into calluses and roughened areas twice a day.

TIRED FOOT SOAK

Soaking your feet in this bath really gives them a much needed break.

> **2 Tbsp. sea salt, finely ground**
> **2 drops rosemary essential oil**
> **1 drop ginger essential oil**

Mix the essential oils into the sea salt. In a basin large enough to hold your feet, place the sea salt mixture. Add warm water and stir to dissolve the sea salt. Place your feet into the water and let them soak for 15-20 minutes. Remove them from the water and dry them thoroughly.

Variation: Substitute one drop of cypress essential oil for the ginger essential oil.

CLEANSING DEODORIZING
FOOT BATH

> **1 cup apple cider vinegar**
> **½ cup dried sage leaves OR 1 cup fresh sage leaves**

In a saucepan heat the apple cider vinegar with the sage leaves added. Simmer covered for 15 minutes then remove from heat. Strain the herbs from the infused vinegar and discard. Allow the vinegar to cool to lukewarm. Place the infused vinegar into a basin large enough to hold your feet, then add warm water. Place your feet into the water and let them soak for 15-20 minutes. Remove them from the water and dry them thoroughly. Apply foot powder afterwards, if desired.

Variations: Substitute ½ cup dried thyme leaves or 1 cup fresh thyme leaves for the sage. OR Substitute ½ cup dried rosemary leaves or 1 cup fresh rosemary leaves for the sage.

Questions and Answers

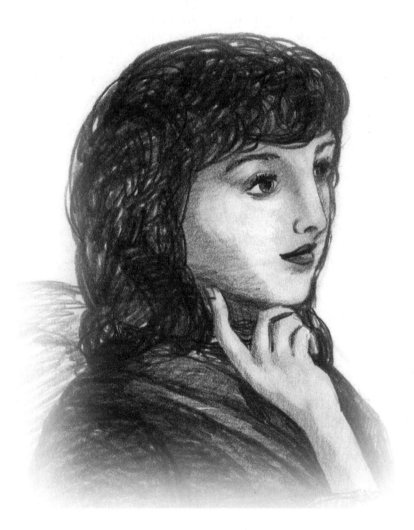

What is and where do you find Turkey Red Oil?

Turkey Red Oil is a specially treated oil (usually castor oil) that will disperse in water without any further treatment. Turkey Red Oil is available through *Lavender Lane*. (See the Resources section of this book.)

When I make hand creams mold growth develops on the surface after a few days. What should I do?

First of all, start with very clean equipment. After melting and combining the ingredients, pour into very clean containers. While the mixture is cooling, cover the product with a layer of paper towel to prevent any airborne molds from contaminating the mixture. Never omit the addition of the natural preservative that is called for in the recipe such as Vitamin E, grapefruit seed extract, and/or tincture of benzoin.

How can I prolong the shelf life of hand creams for long-term storage?

Store the cream in the refrigerator. For longer storage, store the creams in the freezer. To use, thaw the mixture and use as needed.

What are cellulose chips, and where can I find them?

Cellulose chips are usually ground-up corn cobs, although they can be made from other plant materials. They can be found at pet supply stores sold as bedding. *Lavender Lane* carries a product called "Mother Potpourri Magic" that is plant-based and a good fixative for essential oils. (See the Resources section of this book.)

What are sea salts?

They are salts mined from the sea or mined from former sea beds that are located on currently dry ground. Sea salts contain more minerals than common table salt. Sea salts are marketed as sea salts or earth salts. Some sea salts are labeled with the sea where they originated, for example, Dead Sea salts.

Is there a difference between oil and essential oil?

Yes. Oils are derived from nuts, seeds, or fruits. They are often obtained by a procedure called "cold pressing". They are used as carriers for other substances and have an oily feel. Essential oils are not "oils" in the way that is commonly thought. They are derived from various parts of any given plant, usually by steam distillation. Essential oils are diluted for topical use and enhance the body in different ways depending on what plant is used. Pure essential oils have an entirely different makeup than carrier oils, and will not have an oily feel.

I have multiple allergies. Will natural ingredients work for me?

Despite being derived from substances available in nature, natural ingredients can still cause adverse reactions to susceptible people. Persons with sensitivities to multiple substances should seek the advice of an allergist for guidelines on what is safe for them to use. Allergists are physicians specially trained to give help and guidance in these circumstances.

Is there a difference between paraffin and beeswax?

Paraffin is a petroleum byproduct with a waxy consistency. Beeswax is a waxy product produced naturally by honeybees. I recommend using 100% pure beeswax for its natural healing and protective properties.

Why is mineral oil not a good ingredient to have in skin care preparations?

Mineral oil's large molecular structure blocks skin pores and prevents nutrients and essential oils from being absorbed into the skin. It can also prevent wastes from being excreted from the skin pores. The blocking of skin pores over time can lead to permanently enlarged pores.

Can I increase the quantity of products in any of the recipes in this book?

Most of the recipes can be made in a larger quantity without changing the consistency of the finished product. Simply multiply all of the stated ingredients in equal amounts.

I have seen two different kinds of chamomile essential oils. Is there any difference between the two of them and can they be used interchangeably?

There are two kinds of chamomile. One, Roman chamomile or *Anthemis nobilis,* is a perennial herb whose essential oil is a clear yellowish color. The other is German chamomile or *Matricaria recutita,* an annual herb whose essential oil is a deep blue color due to the presence of azulenes in its makeup. Either can be used for skin care, although I prefer the German chamomile essential oil. It seems to have more anti-inflammatory properties due to the high content of azulenes, making it more helpful when used for sensitive and/or troubled skin conditions.

I would like to set up a business and sell homemade cosmetics. How do I go about it?

There are many regulations regarding the making of cosmetics for retail sale. Check the federal laws concerning the manufacture of cosmetics. Also check with your local Board of Health concerning local and state regulations. Have all of the facts and knowledge of the laws that you must follow before attempting to start such a business. Weigh all of the pros and cons, figure in the initial startup costs of starting a business, and truly analyze the reasons why you want to start such a business before you begin. It will save you a lot of backtracking and unexpected expenses if you do your preliminary research.

I purchased some beeswax from my local beekeeper and it has some dark flecks in it. Is it all right to use it?

Your beeswax most likely has small bits of material in it that came out of the hive. They should be removed from the beeswax before you use it. The following method for removing any particles from beeswax was recommended to me by a local beekeeper's wife. I have found that it works very well. Clean several small empty yogurt containers and set aside. Cut a piece of discarded nylon hosiery into a 6 inch square and set aside. Place the beeswax in a clean can with the lid completely removed. Put the can into a saucepan that has 2-3 inches of boiling water in it. Heat the beeswax until it is completely melted. Remove the can of melted beeswax from the boiling water using a hot pad or mitt. Stretch the piece of nylon over the opening of the can and fix it into place with one or two rubber bands. Holding the can with a hot pad or mitt, carefully pour the beeswax into the clean yogurt containers. I usually fill each yogurt container with one to two inches of beeswax. Let the strained beeswax cool until it is solid again, then remove it from the yogurt containers. The cleaned chunks of beeswax usually pop out of the containers easily, but you can cut the containers off if needed. Store the chunks of beeswax in reclosable plastic bags until you are ready to use them.

My normally oily skin becomes very dry during the cold winter months that we have where we live. How should I treat my changeable skin?

Winter weather in many parts of our country bring cold dry air that affects our skin differently. If you find that your skin becomes dry during the winter, use skin care products specifically indicated for dry skin conditions.

I find that I can't use many products because my skin is sensitive and reacts badly to them. What should I do?

Very sensitive skin that reacts to many ingredients should be treated with special care. Extreme caution should be used when applying any new ingredients to your skin. When you have sensitive skin and want to make your own products, introduce any ingredients that you want to use one ingredient at a time. Use a patch test for sensitivity with each ingredient before adding it to any home made product. For multiple sensitivity reactions and continued problems, seek out the advice of a health care professional. They can help guide you through choices of appropriate skin care treatments.

Does Sodium Lauryl Sulfate cause any problems? It is listed as an ingredient on most baby shampoo labels.

Sodium Lauryl Sulfate (SLS) and Sodium Laureth Sulfate (SLES) are common ingredients in shampoos, cosmetic cleaners, toothpastes, and body cleansing gels. Both substances are derived from coconut oil. They are cosmetic detergents and emulsifiers that help to remove oil and dirt from hair and skin. They are the ingredients that give products foaming and bubbling action as well. In clinical studies SLS and SLES have been shown to cause eye irritation and, less frequently, skin irritation in susceptible individuals.

There have rumors circulating over other toxic effects from these ingre-dients but they are only unsubstantiated rumors. There have been no other proven toxic reactions to these ingredients. If you have concerns about using a product with SLS or SLES as ingredients, use liquid castile soap as a substitute. When used as a shampoo, castile soap will leave a film on the hair unless it is followed by a rinse of an acidic substance such as vinegar or lemon juice.

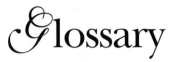

Glossary

Acid Mantle – Body fluid composed of sweat, fresh sebum, and other cell secretions that bathe the surface of the skin. It is thought to act as a natural defense barrier for the skin.

Anti-inflammatory – A substance that counteracts inflammation.

Antioxidant – A substance that blocks or slows oxidation which is a process that produces free radicals, potentially destructive compounds that can cause cell damage.

Antiseptic – A substance that prevents or stops the growth of microorganisms.

Astringent – A substance that causes the skin pores to tighten, increasing the tone of tissues.

Carrier – A substance that is used to transport, dilute, and/or suspend another substance that should not or cannot be applied full strength to the skin. Examples are vegetable oils such as sweet almond, olive, or avocado that are used as carriers for herbs or essential oils.

Cosmetic – A preparation that is made primarily for external use to promote beauty.

Cream – An emulsified cosmetic preparation that usually has a thick consistency.

Decoction – A liquid in which the seeds, roots, or bark of a plant have been simmered in order to extract its active properties.

Dilute – The act of decreasing the concentration of a substance by the addition of another substance.

Dispersible – The ability of an ingredient to be mixed into another substance with even distribution and no separation of the individual ingredients.

Emollient – A substance which, when applied to the skin, softens and smoothes it.

Emulsifier – A substance that enables oily liquids to be dispersed with non-oily liquids.

Extract – A liquid, usually with an alcohol or glycerine base, containing the concentrated properties of an herb which are obtained by a physical or chemical process.

Facial Steam – A process in which the face is placed in an enclosed space, bringing it into contact with hot steam derived from boiling water that is often combined with herbs.

Fixative – A substance that decreases the rapidity of evaporation of essential oils when the two are combined.

Humectant – A substance that promotes the retention of moisture in the skin or draws moisture to the skin.

Infused Oil – A vegetable oil that has selected herbs steeped in it for a given period of time so that the herbal properties are transferred to the oil.

Infusion – A liquid preparation made by adding a selected herb to boiling water and allowing the mixture to steep, dispersing the properties of the herb into the water.

Lotion – A liquid cosmetic preparation that has a slightly thick consistency.

Macerate – The act of softening an herb by soaking or steeping it in a liquid.

Mask – A cosmetic preparation that is applied to the face and left on for a given period of time to achieve effects such as skin softening or toning.

Organic – Plant materials that have been grown without the use of synthetic chemicals, pesticides, and herbicides.

Phototoxic – A substance that is capable of causing an adverse reaction when applied to the skin and then exposed to direct sunlight or a tanning booth session.

Potentiate – The increase in activity of a particular substance when it is used in combination with another specific substance. This activation is selective and does not occur with the combination of all substances.

Preservative – An additive used to slow decay and spoilage of a mixture.

Rancid – A spoiled substance that is no longer useable. Usually a rancid substance has an unpleasant, bitter, or "off" odor. This term is most frequently used when referring to oils or substances that contain oils.

Sebum – A fatty substance secreted by glands in the skin that has a lubricating quality.

Scrub – A coarsely textured mixture gently rubbed on the skin to cleanse deeply.

Tepid – A word that means lukewarm, usually referring to water temperature.

Tincture – A liquid preparation made by steeping herbs in alcohol or glycerine and water to extract their active properties.

Tisane – An infusion of herbs and water that is very similar to a tea.

Topical – A word that describes the external application of any substance.

Toner – A substance that tightens or tones the skin.

Volatile – A characteristic of a substance that describes its ability to vaporize quickly.

*B*ibliography

An asterisk [*] after an entry indicates a book that contains information on herb gardening.

Abehsera, Michel. *The Healing Clay.* New York, NY: Citadel Press, 1990.

Bark, Joseph P., MD *Retin A and Other Youth Miracles.* Rocklin, CA: Prima Publishing and Communication, 1989.

Berwick, Ann. *Holistic Aromatherapy.* St. Paul, MN: Llewellyn Publications, 1994.

Boxer, Arabella and Phillipa Back. *The Herb Book.* New York, NY: Octopus Books Ltd. 1980.

Bricklin, Mark. *Rodale's Encyclopedia of Natural Home Remedies.* Emmaus, PA: Rodale Press, 1982.

Brumberg, Elaine. *Take Care of Your Skin.* New York, NY: Harper & Row Publishers, 1989.

Buchman, Dian Dincin. *Herbal Medicine.* New York, NY: David McKay Co., Inc., 1979.

Byers, Dorie. *Herbal Remedy Gardens.* Pownal, VT. Storey Communications, Inc., 1999.*

Castleman, Michael. *The Healing Herbs.* Emmaus, PA: Rodale Press, 1991.

Cavitch, Susan Miller. *The Natural Soap Book.* Pownal, VT: Storey Communications, Inc., 1995.

Chase, Deborah. *The Medically Based No Nonsense Beauty Book.* New York, NY: Henry Holt & Co., 1989.

Chevalier, Andrew. *The Encyclopedia of Medicinal Plants.* New York, NY: DK Publishing Inc., 1996.

Cooksley, Valerie Gennari. *Aromatherapy, A Lifetime Guide to Healing with Essential Oils.* Englewood Cliffs, NJ: Prentice Hall, 1996.

Damian, Peter & Kate. *Aromatherapy Scent and Psyche.* Rochester, VT: Healing Arts Press, 1995.

Davis, Julie. *Young Skin for Life.* Emmaus, PA: Rodale Press, 1995.

Dodt, Colleen K. *The Essential Oils Book.* Pownal, VT: Storey Communications, Inc., 1996.

Garland, Sarah. *The Complete Book of Herbs and Spices.* London, England: Frances Lincoln Publishers Ltd., 1979.

Gladstar, Rosemary. *Herbal Healing for Women.* New York, NY: Simon & Schuster, 1993.

Greig, Denise. *The Complete Book of Potpourri and Perfumery*. Kenthurst, New South Wales, Australia: Kangaroo Press, 1992.

Jacobs, Betty M. *Growing and Using Herbs Successfully*. Pownal, VT: Storey Communications, Inc., 1981.*

Kanner, Catherine. *Beauty from a Country Garden*. Berkley, CA: Ten Speed Press, 1992.

Kowalchik, Claire and William H. Hylton, Editors. *Rodale's Illustrated Encyclopedia of Herbs*. Emmaus, PA: Rodale Press, 1987.*

Lawless, Julia. *The Illustrated Encyclopedia of Essential Oils*. New York, NY: Barnes & Noble Books, 1995.

MacKie, Rona M. *Healthy Skin—The Facts*. Oxford, England: Oxford University Press, 1992.

McClure, Susan. *The Herb Gardener: A Guide for All Seasons*. Storey Communications, Inc., 1996.*

McIntyre, Anne. *The Complete Woman's Herbal*. New York, NY: Henry Holt Co., 1994.

Mills, Simon Y. *Out of the Earth*. New York, NY: Penguin Books, 1991.

Ody, Penelope. *The Complete Medicinal Herbal*. New York, NY: DK Publishing, Inc., 1993.

Rose, Jeanne. *The Aromatherapy Book*. Berkley, CA: North Atlantic Books, 1992.

Rose, Jeanne. *Herbs and Things: Jeanne Rose's Herbal*. New York, NY: Perigee Books, 1972.

Ryman, Daniele. *Aromatherapy—The Complete Guide to Plant and Flower Essences for Health and Beauty*. New York, NY: Bantam Books, 1993.

Schoen, Linda Allen, Editor. *The AMA Book of Skin and Hair Care*. Philadelphia, PA: J.P. Lippincott Co., 1976.

Serrentino, Jo. *How Natural Remedies Work*. Point Roberts, WA: Hartley & Marks Inc., 1991.

Stuart, Malcolm, Editor. *The Encyclopedia of Herbs and Herbalism*. New York, NY: Crescent Publishing, 1987.*

Tolley, Emelie and Chris Mead. *Gifts from the Herb Garden*. New York, NY: Clarkson Potter Publishers, Inc., 1991.

Westerman, Kaila. *Melt and Mold Soapmaking*. Pownal, VT: Storey Communications, Inc., 2000.

Worwood, Valerie Ann. *The Complete Book of Essential Oils and Aromatherapy*.

Resources

Look for ingredients locally in natural or health food stores. If you can't find them there, here is a list of companies that offer a wide variety of ingredients and supplies for sale. Check with each individual company regarding the availability of catalogues.

Clays, Essential Oils, Oils, Earth Salts, D-Panthenol, Aloe Vera Gel, and Other Ingredients

THE FRUITFUL YIELD DIRECT
Bloomingdale, IL
1-800-469-5552

Oils, Essential Oils, Containers, Turkey Red Oil, Beeswax, Mother Potpourri Magic (Cellulose Chips), and Other Ingredients

LAVENDER LANE, INC.
P.O. Box 600
Merlin, OR 97532
Phone: 888-593-4400

Website: www.lavenderlane.com

Oils, Essential Oils, Beeswax, Herbs, and Other Ingredients

HERBAL HEALER ACADEMY, INC.
HC32, 97-B
Mt. View, AR 72560
Phone: 870-269-4177
Fax: 1-800-76-FAXUS
Website: www.herbalhealer.com

Herbs, Clay, Beeswax, Oils, Containers, Aura Cacia and Frontier Essential Oils, and Other Ingredients

FRONTIER NATURAL PRODUCTS COOPERATIVE
3021 78th St.
PO Box 299
Norway, IA 52318
Phone: 1-800-669-3275
Website: www.frontiercoop.com

Oils, Essential Oils, Soap Molds, Soapmaking Supplies, Rebatchable Soap Curls, Liquid Soap, Beeswax, and Other Ingredients and Supplies

TKB TRADING, LLC
Kaila Westerman, President
356 24th Street
Oakland, CA 94612
Phone: 510-451-9011
Fax: 510-839-9967
Websites: www.tkbtrading.com, www.alphabetsoap.com

Essential Oils, Oils, Soap Molds, Beeswax, Liquid Soap, Containers, Rebatchable Soap Curls, Soapmaking Supplies, Super Silk, and Other Ingredients and Supplies

JANE'S SMALL GIFTS
(Authorized Distributor of TKB Trading)
PO Box 32126
Mesa, AZ 85275-2126
Phone: 430-835-1634
Website: www.janessmallgifts.com
E-mail: soap@janessmallgifts.com

100% Pure Essential Oils, Beeswax, Floral Waxes, Dead Sea Salts, Soapmaking Supplies, Hydrosols, Exotic Oils and Butters, Botanicals, Soap Molds, Containers, and Other Ingredients and Supplies

RAINBOW MEADOW
PO Box 457
Napoleon, MI 49261
Phone: 1-800-207-4047 or 517-764-9795
Fax: 517-764-0940
Website: www.rainbowmeadow.com
E-mail: info@rainbow.com

Wholesale Ingredients, Information on Retailers of Their Products (NOW Foods Sells Organic Essential Oils, Oils, Clays, Earth Salts, D-Panthenol, Aloe Vera Gel, and Other Ingredients.)

NOW NATURAL FOODS
395 South Glen Ellyn Rd.
Bloomingdale, IL 60108
Phone: 1-800-999-8069
Website: www.nowfoods.com
E-mail: sales@nowfoods.com

Dr. Bronner's Magic Soaps (Liquid and Bar Castile Soaps)

The staff at Dr. Bronner's recommends that you purchase their products
through a local health food store. For information on their products
and other health related information:
DR. BRONNER'S MAGIC SOAPS
PO Box 28
Escondido, CA 92033
Phone: 760-743-2211
Website: www.drbronner.com

Containers and Bottles of All Kinds

SKS BOTTLING AND PACKAGING
3 Knabner Rd.
Mechanicville, NY 12118
Phone: 518-899-7488
Fax: 1-800-810-0440
Website: www.sks-bottle.com
E-mail: sales@sks-bottle.com

Containers and Bottles of All Kinds

SUNBURST BOTTLE CO.
5710 Auburn Blvd. Ste 7
Sacramento, CA 95841
Phone: 916-348-5576
Fax: 916-348-3803
Website: www.sunburstbottle.com
E-mail: sunburst@cwo.com

Glass, Plastic, and Metal Packaging and Closures

BURCH BOTTLE & PACKAGING INC.
811 Tenth St.
Watervliet, NY 12189
Phone: 1-800-903-2830 or 518-273-1846
Fax: 518-273-1846
Website: www.burchbottle.com
(Please call, fax, write, or visit the company's website to request a free catalogue.)

All Natural Sunscreens, Sun Care Products, and Natural Body Care Products for Adults and Babies

BRONZO SENSUALÉ
1020 Stillwater Dr.
Miami Beach, FL 33141
Phone: 1-800-991-2226
Fax: 305-867-1745
Website: www.bronzosensuale.com
E-mail: suntan@bronzosensuale.com

$\mathcal{I}$ndex

Check Out These Other Vital Health Titles!

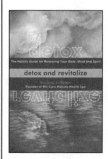
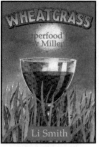
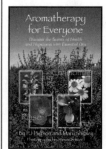
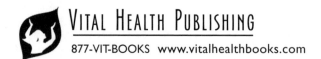